ENCYCLOPAEDIA OF
TISSUE CULTURE

Encyclopaedia of
Tissue Culture

Volume 1

M.S. Ahmad

ANMOL PUBLICATIONS PVT. LTD.
NEW DELHI - 110 002 (INDIA)

ANMOL PUBLICATIONS PVT. LTD.
H.O.: 4374/4B, Ansari Road, Darya Ganj,
New Delhi-110 002 (India)
Ph.: 23278000, 23261597
B.O.: No. 1015, Ist Main Road, BSK IIIrd Stage
IIIrd Phase, IIIrd Block
Bangalore - 560 085 (India)
Visit us at: www.anmolpublications.com

Encyclopaedia of Tissue Culture

First Published, 2007

ISBN 81-261-3084-9 (Set)

PRINTED IN INDIA

Printed at Mehra Offset Press, Delhi.

Contents

Preface

A cell is the smallest unit of the body of a living or non-living object. And a combination of cells is called 'tissue'. Tissues are of different kinds and of different shapes and sizes. Some are cylindrical; some are circular; some are long and some others are short in length. Besides, some are soft; some are medium and hard. In common parlance, they form the flesh, blood and bones.

With the advancement in Science and Technology, experiments were also made in this branch of Biology. Replacement of tissues is the major thrust area. Plastic surgery is an example in this connection. With the help of this technology, faces can be changed to any extent. This technology has proved to be a boon for the victims of fire or terrorist attacks.

Like animals, plant tissues also hold a great importance. New to newer experiments are being made at different botanical labs to increase the produce of hybrid plants of varied characteristics. It is a bright career-field and a lot has yet to be done in future.

Encyclopaedia of Tissue Culture attempts at bringing all the relevant and uptodate information on this subject. This multi-volume work includes various aspects of tissue culture at length. Students, scholars, academics, doctors and the general readers would find it equally useful and beneficial.

Comments and suggestions sent by sincere readers would be of great importance to us.

— Editor

1

Introduction

The development of specialised cell types from a single fertilized egg cell is called differentiation (see Table). The cell differentiation involves changes in biochemistry and function of the cell and is preceded by commitment of the cell to a particular fate. Therefore, cell commitment and cell differentiation are two different steps in the development of specialised cell types. The cell commitment has also been divided into specification and determination.

The cell is specified when it differentiates autonomously, only if placed in a neutral environment, but is said to be determined if it becomes capable of differentiating autonomously even when placed in another environment (in another region of the embryo, *e.g.* by transplantation). Specification followed by determination leads to irreversible commitment. Usually a cell becomes determined before it differentiates, although in some cases the two processes occur simultaneously. Sometimes, it is also possible for the differentiation to occur without determination, but this differentiation is often reversible. A brief account of different forms of cell commitment (involving specification and determination) and the mechanism involved in this commitment.

There are three major ways known for cell commitment, which are briefly outlined in Table.

(i) Autonomous specification involves specificity due to the cell's own internal cytoplasmic components acquired due to segregation of these cytoplasmic components during embryonic cleavage; this is also described as *'mosaic development'*.

(ii) Conditional specification involves cells which are capable of following more than one fates depending upon the interactions with the neighbouring cells; this is also described as *'regulative development'*.

(iii) Syncytial specification involves cells whose fates are decided even before the cells are formed due to segregation and interactions between cell components of a multinucleate cell or a syncytium before the nuclei are separated by the membrane.

In most invertebrates, autonomous specification is predominant. In vertebrates, conditional specification is extensively used and in many insects (*e.g. Drosophila)* syncytial specification is witnessed. The differentiation of germ cells is an important subject of cell differentiation.

Autonomous Specifications Determination

Tunicate Embryos: In tunicates, at the time of fertilization, the fertilized egg has been shown to have cytoplasm differentiated into several regions destined to give rise to different kinds of cells. As the fertilized egg divides, different resulting cells (also called blastomeres) incorporate different cytoplasmic regions, which are believed to contain morphogenetic determinants (Fig.). The different regions of cytoplasm can be visualised by their different colours and become apportioned into various blastomeres. The first division cleaves the egg into right and left mirror images and both sides then undergo similar cell divisions. Each coloured region gives rise to a different part as follows:

Some Differentiated Cell Types in Animal Systems and their Major Products (from Gilbert, 1994)

	Cell Type	Differentiated cell product	Specialised function
1.	Keratinocyte (skin cell)	Keratin	Protection against abrasion, desiccation
2.	Erythrocyte (red blood cell)	Haemoglobin	Transport of oxygen
3.	Lens cell	Crystallins	Transmission of light
4.	B lymphocyte	Immunoglobulins	Antibody synthesis
5.	T lymphocyte	Cell surface antigens (lymphokines)	Destruction of foreign cells; regulation of immune response
6.	Melanocyte	Melanin	Pigment production
7.	Pancreatic islet cells Insulin	Regulation of carbohydrate metabolism	
8.	Leydig cell (♂) Testosterone	Male sexual characteristics	
9.	Chondrocyte (cartilage cell)	Chondroitin sulfate; type II collagen	Tendons and ligaments
10.	Osteoblast (bone-forming cell)	Bone matrix	Skeletal support
11.	Myocyte (muscle cell)	Muscle actin and myosin	Contraction
12.	Hepatocyte (liver cell)	Serum albumin; numerous enzymes	Production of serum proteins and numerous enzymatic functions
13.	Neurons	Neurotransmitters (acetylcholine, epinephrine, etc.)	Transmission of electrical impulses
14.	Tubule cell (♀) of hen oviduct	Ovalbumin	Egg white proteins
15.	Follicle cel (♀) of insect oviduct	Chorion proteins	Egg shell proteins

(i) the yellow cytoplasmic crescent gives rise to the muscle cells;

(ii) the grey equatorial crescent produces the notochord cytoplasm and the neural tube;

(iii) the clear animal cytoplasm becomes the larval epidermis and

(iv) the yolky grey vegetal region gives rise to the larval gut. In an experiment conducted in 1940s, it was shown that if from an 8-celled embryo, four pairs of blastomeres are separated and allowed to develop, they develop into separate specific structures showing autonomous cell specification (Fig.).

Later in 1970s, biochemical confirmation of cytoplasmic segregation of tissue determinants became available. For instance, one pair of cells from 8-celled embryo was capable of producing tail muscle and they only stained positively for the presence of acetylcholinesterase suggesting that this enzyme has something to do with the specificity of these cells to form tail muscles.

The autonomous determination is accomplished by two types of mechanisms at the molecular level; (i) the first mechanism involves localisation and partitioning of factors like transcription factors which activate transcription of specific genes like that for acetylcholinesterase. In such cases, treatment with actinomycin D (transcription inhibitor) will allow no transcription of this gene, but fresh supply of mRNA allows the production of the protein suggesting that only transcription activation is involved. (ii) The second mechanism involves localisation and partitioning of the messages and proteins that are characteristic of a cell type. An example is the synthesis of intestinal alkaline phosphatase. This enzyme is synthesized by the larval endoderm leading to the segregation of cell types forming the gut in the tunicate embryo.

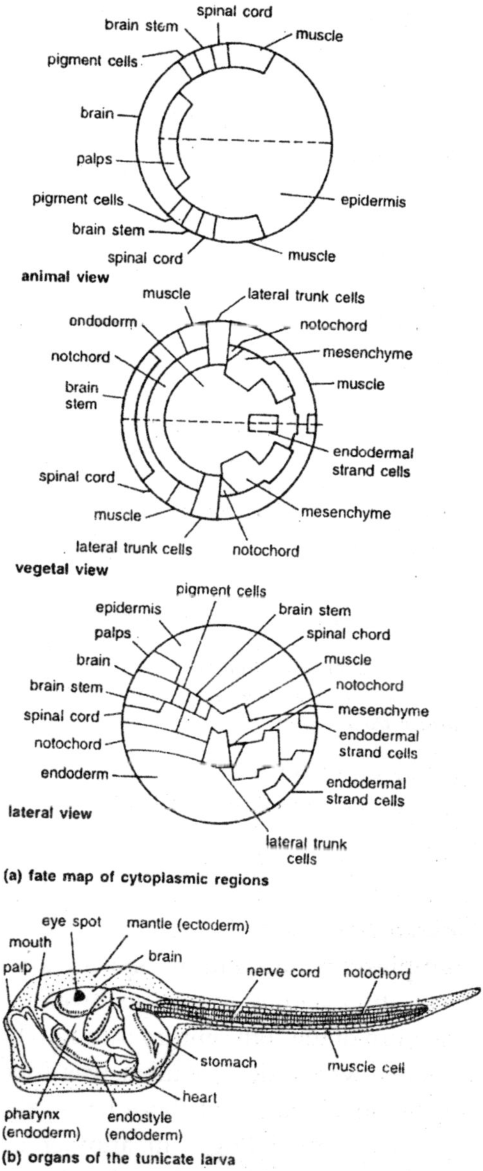

Segregation of cytoplasmic determinants at the time of fertilization in tunicate Phallusia mammillata. (a) three views of the fate map; (b) the organs of tunicate larva. (redrawn from Gilbert 'Developmental Biology', 1994).

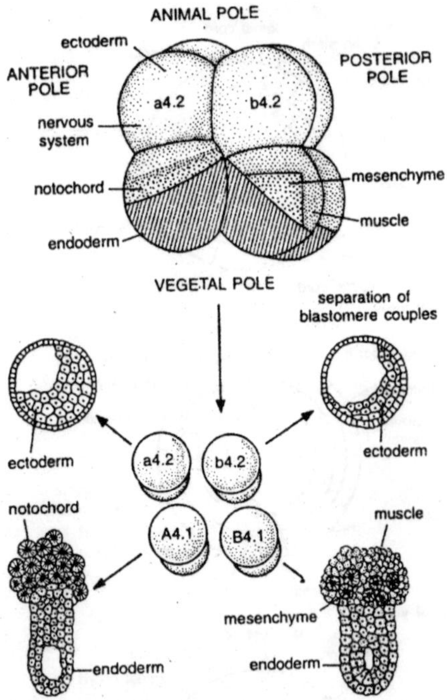

Mosaic determination in tunicates, from an 8-celled embryo; when four blastomere couples are dissociated, they develop into different structures, as shown (redrawn from Gilbert 'Developmental Biology', 1994).

Actinomycin D has no effect on synthesis of enzyme in this case, but the inhibitors of translation prevent such a synthesis. This suggests that mRNA must pre-exist in these cells and that the regulation is exercised only at the translational level.

Mollusc Embryo: Molluscs (*e.g. Patella coerulea)* also provide interesting examples of autonomous specification due to cytoplasmic localisation leading to mosaic development. This was proved at the turn of the 20th century through the isolation of early blastomeres, whose development was followed and compared with the development of those left in the embryo. No difference was observed (Fig.). In another experiment involving spirally cleaving embryos (some molluscs and some annelids), where a polar lobe is formed, the lobe was shown to have mesodermal determinants for the development of

Modes of Cell Type Specification and their Characteristics

I. Autonomous Specification

A characteristic of most invertebrates; specification by acquisition of certain cytoplasmic molecules present in the egg; invariant cleavages produce the same lineages in each embryo of the species; blastomere fates are generally invariant; lineage "founder cells" are usually specified autonomously at poles of embryonic axes; cell type specification precedes any large-scale embryonic cell migration; produces 'mosaic' ('determinative') development: cells cannot change fate if a blastomere is lost.

II. Conditional Specification

Characteristic of all vertebrates and few invertebrates; specification by interactions between cells; relative positions are important; variable cleavages produce no invariant fate assignments to cells; massive cell rearrangements and migrations precede or accompany specification; capacity for "regulative" development; allows cells to acquire different functions.

III. Syncytial Specification

Characteristic of most insect classes; specification of body regions by interactions between cytoplasmic regions prior to cellularisation of the blastoderm; variable cleavage produces no rigid cell fates for particular nuclei; after cellularisation, conditional specification is most often seen.

Source: *Modified from Davidson, 1991.*

mesodermal organs (muscles, mouth, shell gland and foot). These determinants were later shown to be located in the cytoskeleton and not in the diffusible cytoplasm. The determinants in the polar lobe actually control the following:

(i) proper rhythm and cleavage orientation of the D blastomere,

(ii) mesodermal and intestinal differentiation,

(iii) inductive interaction and

(iv) specification of dorsal-ventral axis of the embryo.

Coenorhabditis Elegans Embryo: *Coenorhabditis elegans* is a small (1 mm long) free living soil nematode, which has rapid period (about 16 hours) of embryogenesis giving rise to 1090 somatic cells in the hermaphrodite. These 1090 cells belonged to only few cell types. The predominant form of this organism is hermaphrodite and males are infrequent (no females are known). They reproduce either by self fertilization or by cross fertilization (⚥ × ♂).

The body is covered by a transparent cuticle, so that the development can be followed by observations in a Petri dish. Entire lineage of 1090 cells has been mapped by such observations through transparent cuticle. These features made this organism to be the choice for study of cell biology and development biology.

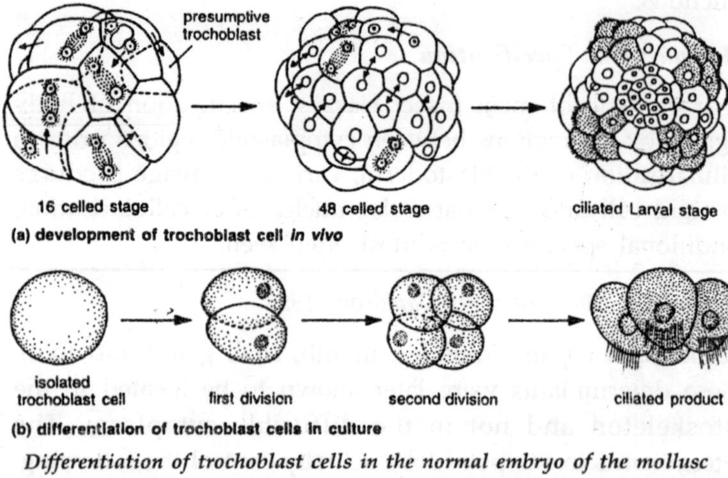

Differentiation of trochoblast cells in the normal embryo of the mollusc Patella; both in vivo, as well as in vitro (isolated cells), trochoblast cells become ciliated at the correct time (redrawn from Gilbert 'Developmental Biology', 1994).

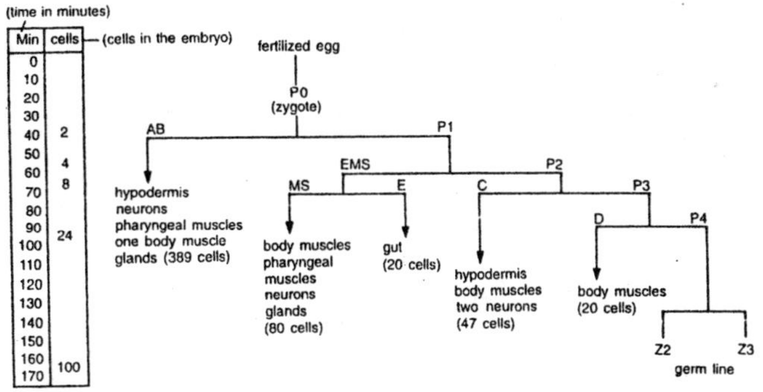

Abbreviated cell lineage chart for Coenorhabditis elegans, emphasising the germ line precursors (P cells, P0-P4), that receive the P granules (redrawn from Gilbert 'Developmental Biology', 1994).

The animal has six pairs of chromosomes. It has 1500-3000 essential genes and over 10,000 non-essential genes. This is a very small number of genes for a multicellular organism. The haploid genome has 10^8 base pairs of DNA, about the same as in *Drosophila.* The first four asymmetric and asynchronous cell divisions, each produces one 'differentiating' daughter cell (they are called founder cells) and another stem cell. In this manner five founder cells (AB, MS, E, C, D) and four stem cells (P_1, P_2, P_3, P_4) are produced (Fig.). These asymmetric cell divisions are associated with asymmetric localisation of cytoplasmic substances into specific blastomeres. In the egg and zygote are found germ line granules or P granules, which later become restricted to the posterior cytoplasmic region forming cells that are capable of forming gametes. The blastomeres P_1, P_2, P_3 and P_4 will contain the granules and the founder cells (AB, MS, E, C, D) will lack these granules. Such localisation of the granules is facilitated by microfilaments but no microtubules are needed. Six *par* (partitioning defective) genes control cytoplasmic partitioning in one cell zygote to create anterior-posterior polarity.

However, P granules do not enter the nucleus and their role in development is unknown. Another maternally inherited protein called skn-1 protein (product of *skn-1* gene) may function as a transcription factor and activate genes in the

P_1 cell and its descendants. There are two other genes *(pie-1* and *mex-1),* mutations in alter the determination of cells in the 8-cell embryo. It is hypothesized that the products of these two genes are required to either localise or regulate the wild type *skn-1* gene product.

Dependent Specification

In sea urchin (a deuterosome) and the vertebrates, during embryo development the fate of a cell depends either on (i) who its ancestral cells, were? or on (ii) who its neighbouring cells are? In the latter case, each cell starts off with similar potential and develops according to whom it meets. In these embryos, upto a certain stage, each cell is able to develop into the entire embryo, if it is separated from other cells. This type of conditional specification or regulative development is different from autonomous specification discussed earlier, where the cytoplasmic determinats played a major role in determining the fate of the cell. The phenomenon of identical twins in mammals like human beings also suggests regulative development of embryos.

The foundation experiments demonstrating regulative development were first conducted by Hans Driesch, as early as 1892. He isolated sea urchin blastomeres from each other

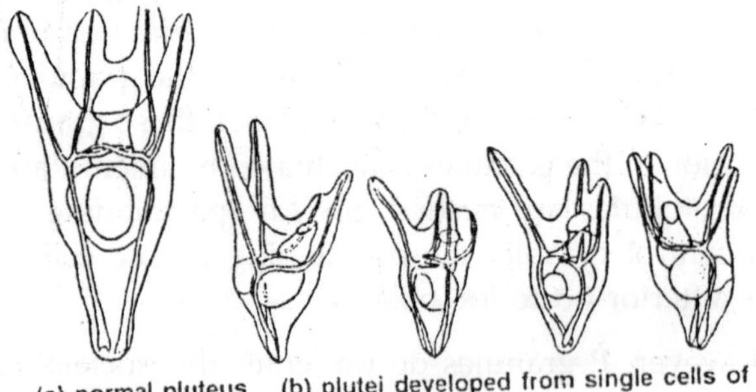

Regulative development of sea urchin larva, where individual blastomeres were separated at four celled stage and were allowed to develop; the blastomeres gave smaller, but normal plutei; compare size in (a) and (b), (redrawn from Gilbert 'Developmental Biology', 1994).

by vigorous shaking and found that each blastomere from a 2-8 cell embryo developed into a complete larva. This was the first experimental evidence of regulative development, where each blastomere could regulate its development to produce a complete organism. Driesch later concluded that the development proceeded by interactions between the nucleus and the cytoplasm and that for an isolated blastomere, the 'prospective potency' (the cell types, that were possible to be formed by it) was greater than its 'prospective fate' (the cell that it would normally form).

In a series of experiments conducted later by Sven Horstadius, it was shown that the sea urchin embryo is not a mere collection of completely equipotential cells. For instance, when 8 cell embryo (or even an unfertilized egg) was divided meridionally through both animal and vegetal poles, both halves produced larvae as observed by Driesch, but when it was divided equatorially (separating animal and vegetal poles), neither part developed into a complete larva, the animal half becoming a hollow ball of ciliated epidermal cells (called dauerblastula) and the vegetal half developing into an abnormal larva (Fig.). These experiments suggested that the determinants that enable micromere formation and gastrulation resided in the vegetal portion.

Horstadius, later conducted experiments to study the fate of each of the six tiers of cells in 64 cell sea urchin embryo and demonstrated that:

(i) animal layer and the first vegetal layer normally produce ectoderm,

(ii) the second vegetal layer gives rise to endoderm and some larval mesoderm and

(iii) the micromeres generate the mesodermal skeleton.

However, when the tiers were separated and recombined in various ways, the original fates of these tiers were altered

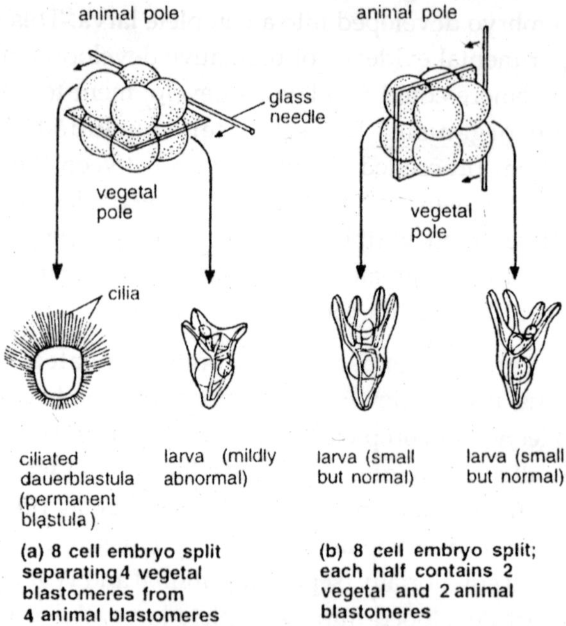

Early asymmetry in the sea urchin embryo, showing that both animal and vegetal blastomeres are needed for the development of normal larva. (a) when animal blastomeres are separated from vegetal blastomeres, the former develop into dauerblastula and the latter into a slightly abnormal larva; (b) when each half contains animal and vegetal blastomeres, small, but normal appearing larvae develop (redrawn from Gilbert 'Developmental Biology', 1994).

by the new neighbours, thus suggesting a regulative development. In another set of experiments, when micromeres from the vegetal pole were transplanted into the animal cap of 16 cell sea urchin embryo, these cells induced the formation of archenteron by the animal cap cells, although normally archenteron is formed on the vegetal side (Fig.). This again suggested that neighbouring cells (micromeres), may send signals changing the fate of animal cap cells.

Organiser and Primary Embryonic Induction: The above discussion shows that in sea urchin and vertebrates, although individual cells have the potential to develop into a whole organism, till the embryo reaches a certain stage, but its fate

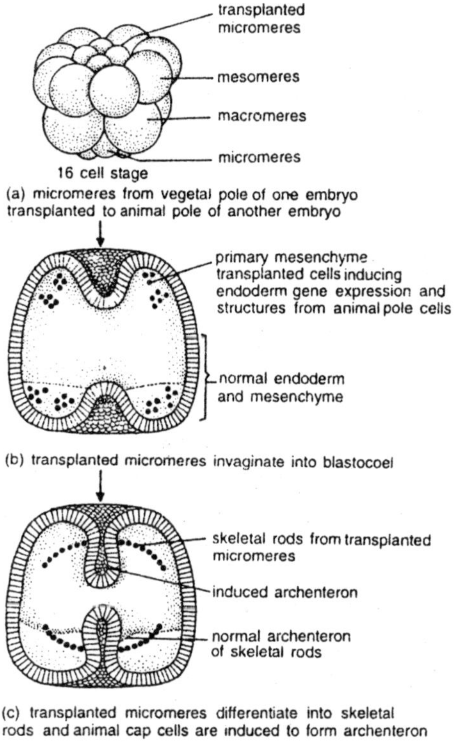

The effect of transplanting fluorescently-labelled micromeres from the vegetal pole of one embryo to the animal pole of another embryo (redrawn from Gilbert 'Developmental Biology', 1994).

is regulated by the nature of the neighbouring cells. This regulation is exercised by restricting the potency of cells by their neighbouring cells. In most cases, cells from one layer restricts the ability of a cell from another layer to express its full potential (Fig.). However, eventually, the blastomeres become committed to certain fates as shown in transplantation experiments summarised in Table. One of the examples of these committed cells is the dorsal blastopore lip cells, which if transplanted, continue to remain as blastopore lip, and initiate gastrulation and embryogenesis in the surrounding tissue at the new transplanted location. It also initiates development of a complete neural plate at the new location in the host tissue thus forming a new embryo, face to face with its host (Fig.). In view of this, the blastopore lip cells are referred to as organiser and the process due to which the fate of one tissue is determined by another tissue is generally called induction. The specific induction, where blastopore lip cells induce dorsal axis and the neural tube is called 'primary embryonic induction'. The organiser not only induces the neural tube, but also specifies the regions of the neural tube, thus determining regional differences.

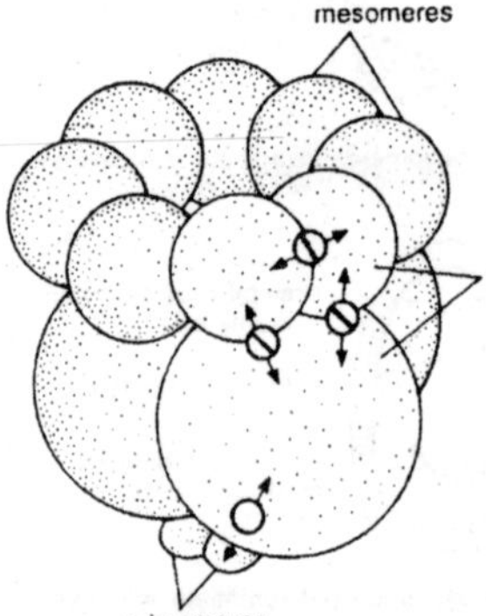

Inhibitory induction in the sea urchin blastula (double headed arrows indicate mutually restrctive interactions (redrawn from Gilbert 'Developmental Biology', 1994).

Results of Tissue Transplantation during Early- and late-gastrula Stages in the Newt as Studied by Hans Spemann (who won Nobel Prize in 1935)

Donor region	*Host region*	*Differentiation of donor tissue*	*Nature of development*
I Early gastrula			
(a) Prospective neurons	Prospective epidermis	Epidermis	Dependent (conditional)
(b) Prospective epidermis	Prospective neurons	Neurons	Dependent (conditional)
II Late gastrula			
(a) Prospective neurons (autonomous)	Prospective epidermis	Neurons	Independent
(b) Prospective epidermis (autonomous)	Prospective neurons	Epidermis	Independent

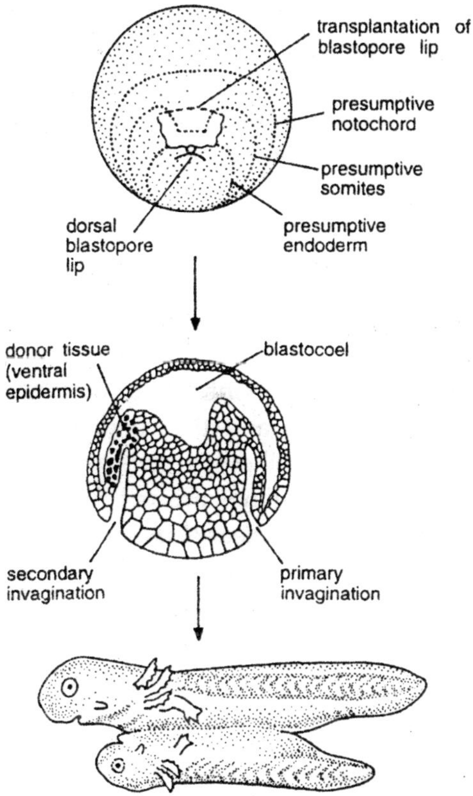

Self differentiation of 'dorsal lip' tissue, as demonstrated by transplantation of dorsal blastopore lip from one early gastrula into another early gastrula, in the region that normally becomes ventral epidermis; tissue invaginates and forms a second archenteron and second embryonic axis (redrawn from Gilbert 'Developmental Biology', 1994).

Competence and Secondary Induction: The primary embryonic induction initiates a cascade of inductive events, by which one tissue interacts with another to specifically directs its fate. These inductive events are described as secondary induction. While the tissue making the 'organiser' produces inducing stimulus, there are tissues that need to respond. This ability to respond in a specific manner to a given stimulus is called competence. For instance, in early gastrula, ectoderm in all regions of the embryo has the competence to form a new neural plate and embryonic axis, but with increasing embryonic age, the ectoderm loses its ability to respond. In other words, at the later stages, the ectoderm loses its competence to respond to new blastopore lip, although it can now respond to new inducers.

Committed Specification

In the previous two sections of this Chapter, we described the autonomous specification (where the cytoplasmic determinants play an important role in determining the fate of early embryonic cells) and the conditional specification (where the position of a cell determines its fate). However, in *Drosophila,* the cell membranes are not formed between the nuclei until after the 13th nuclear division. The nuclei therefore share a common cytoplasm till this 13th division. Therefore, in these insect embryos, the specification of cell types along anterior-posterior and dorsal-ventral axes is achieved by the interactions of cytoplasmic materials within the single multinucleate cell.

In the syncytial blastoderm, during the 9th division cycle, about five nuclei reach the surface of the posterior pole of the embryo. Three nuclei become enclosed in cell membranes and generate the pole cells that give rise to gametes. Most of the other nuclei arrive at the periphery of the embryo at 10th division cycle and then undergo four more divisions. Following 13th division cycle, cell membranes grow between the nuclei to form a cellular blastoderm of about 6000 cells. At 14th division cycle, the level of transcription increases dramatically, cells become motile and the embryo (which is 2-3 hour old) begins gastrulation. At this stage after cellularisation, conditional specification discussed earlier starts operating.

2

Concept and Perception

Principle of Cell

Discovery of Cell and the Cell Theory: All animals and plants consist of certain structural units. Such a concept was originally put forward by Aristotle (384-322 B.C.). Many centuries later, for these units, a term cell (Gr., kytos, cell; L., cella, hollow space) was used by Robert Hooke, who in 1665, observed these so called cells for the first time in a piece of cork under a very primitive microscope. Later, cells in the form of cavities with cellulose walls were observed in different plants by Grew and Malpighi. In 1674, Leeuwenhoek also discovered free cells and observed some organisation within these cells.

The structural unit called cell, is now known as the unit of life and the concept that the cell is basic unit of life is known as the cell theory. Although at the beginning of 19th century (1802-1826), several workers including a Frenchman, H.J. Dutrochet gave the idea of the cell theory, the credit for formulating the cell theory is normally given to a German botanist, M. I. Schleiden and a German zoologist, T. Schwann who clearly outlined the basic features of the theory in 1839.

However, Schleiden and Schwann only took the old ideas and presented them in the form of a concrete theory. It is suggested, therefore, that the cell theory of Schleiden and Schwann was more an act of synthesis rather than of a discovery.

R. Virchow, in 1858 extended the cell theory and suggested that an additional feature of the cell theory should be that all living cells arise from preexisting living cells. This was important because prior to this realisation there was a belief in the spontaneous creation of life. Later, Louis Pasteur, in France gave experimental evidence to support Virchow's extension of the cell theory.

It is obvious thus, that there are two main components of the cell theory- (i) that living things are composed of cells and (ii) that all cells arise from preexisting cells. Living things, therefore, can be defined as those objects, which are composed of cells capable of reproducing.

In recent years, large number of sub-cellular structures have been discovered and studied in detail. Consequently, it may appear that cell is no longer a basic unit of life, because life may exist without cells also. It should, however; be realised that the importance of the atomic theory in physics and chemistry did not decrease with the discovery of smaller particles like protons, neutrons and electrons. In the same way, although the details of ultrastructure of the cell are now known, showing that it is a very complex structure, the cell theory still remains a very useful concept.

Exceptions to the Cell Theory

A special difficulty is faced when we apply the concept of 'cell theory' to viruses (Fig.) Virus may be defined as an infectious, subcellular and ultramicroscopic particle representing potentially pathogenic agents, whose replication in the host cell and transmission by infection causes characteristic reaction in the host cells. Besides animal and plant viruses, there is another class of viruses, the bacterial

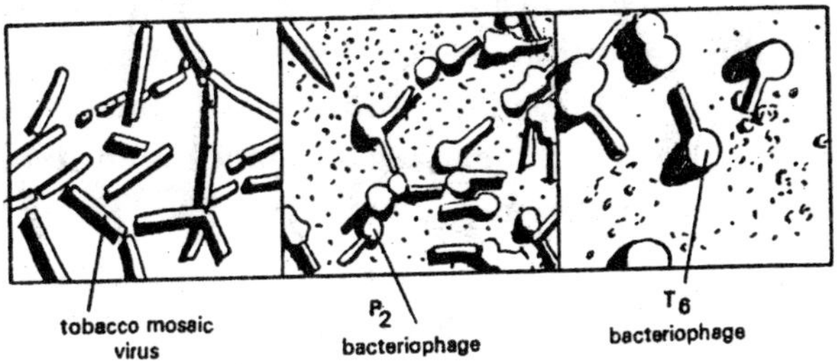

Three different kinds of viruses as seen with the help electron microscope (redrawn from Swanson: The Cell, 1971).

viruses known as bacteriophages (Fig.). In all these cases viruses are so minute that they cannot be visible without the aid of electron microscope. They are also simple so that they lack the internal organisation which is so characteristic of a cell.

Outside the cell, they are just like non-living inert particles. Due to these properties, viruses, do not easily fit in the definition of a cell and they are often described as "living chemicals" or as "cellular" forms that have degenerated through parasitism or "primitive organisms, that have not reacted a cellular state". However, a biologist treats them as if they were individual cells.

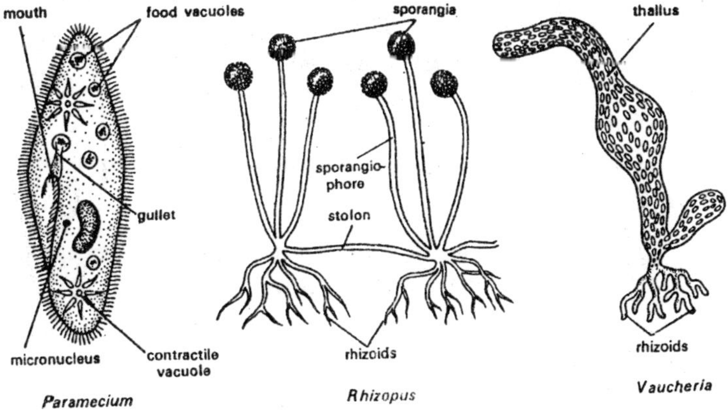

Three cases of acellular organisation (redrawn from Swanson: The Cell, 1971).

There are other organisms in protozoa and algae which do not fit in the definition of cell theory. For instance, in Paramecium, a protozoan, in Rhizopus a fungus and in Vaucheria an alga (Fig.), the living substance is enclosed in a wall and there is hardly any organisation like that of a cell.

Whether cell is a basic unit of structure in these cases? The cases discussed here may r may not be regarded as exceptions to the cell the c but it is difficult to explain their organisation in context of the cell theory.

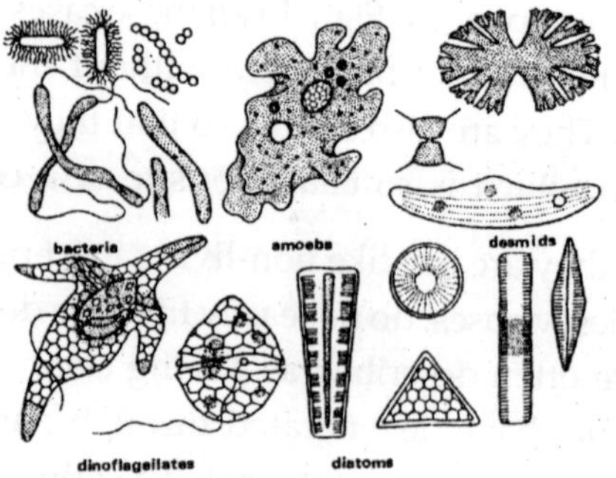

Variety of organisms showing different cell shapes.

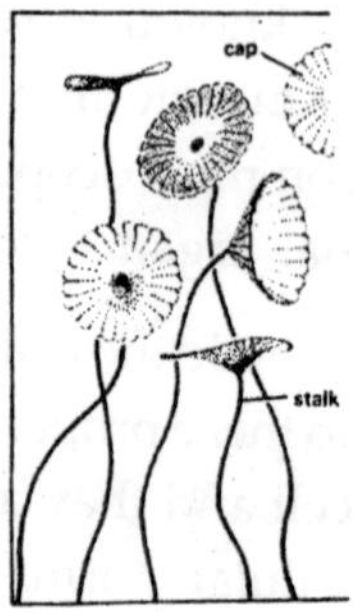

Acetabularia, a single-cell

Shape, Size and Number of Cell

Cell Shape: There is a great amount of variability in cells with respect to the cell shape. Some cells like amoebae and leukocytes change their shapes frequently. Other cells have a typical shape. For instance, some bacteria are rods, spirals and even comas.

Various algae like diatoms and desmids take up varied shapes (Fig.). Another important single-celled alga is Acetabularia, which consists of a stalk and a cap making up to 10 cm in height (Fig.).

The cell size also depends in many cases on the size and the number of chromosomes. In many cases it has been proved that when the chromosome number is artificially doubled, the cell size is automatically increased (Fig.).

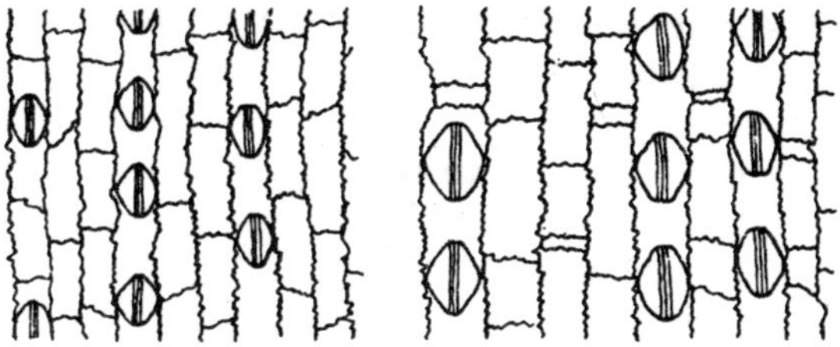

Difference in cell size (stomata) due to difference in ploidy level.

It has also been emphasised that the cell size remains constant during evolution, while other characters may change. One of the possible reasons for this could be that when the cell size increases, the increase in the volume of the cell is much more than the area of cell surface (volume increases as cube of radius, while surface area increases as square of radius).

Due to disproportionate increase in cell volume and surface area, adequate area for exchange of material for the increased volume may not be available. It is for this reason that metabolically active cells, tend to be smaller in size.

In human body, with the exception of some nerve cells, the cell volume ranges from 200 μ^3 to 1,5000 μ^3. In general the cell volume is constant for a cell type and does not depend on the organism. For instance, kidney cells in bull, horse or mouse are of same size and the difference in size of organisms depends on cell number only. This is sometimes called the law of constant volume.

Cell Number: The cell number in an organism also varies from a single cell in a unicellular organism to 60 thousand billion cells in a human being weighing about 80 kg. This number would be more in certain other organisms.

The number of cells in most multicellular organisms is rather indefinite, but it may be fixed in organisms like Pandorina and Eudorina (both green algae), the former with a colony consisting of 8, 16 or 32 or 64 cells and the latter with a colony of 16, 32 or 64 cells.

Prokaryotic Cells and Eukaryotic Cells

Till recently, in living organisms, two types of cells were recognised, prokaryotic cells with no organised nuclei and eukaryotic cells having organised nuclei with nuclear envelopes. The prokaryotes included bacteria and blue green algae, while the eukaryotes included higher organisms (Table).

However, another group of living organisms, the "archaea" was discovered in 1977 and the organisms of this group were described as archaebacteria, so that the prokaroytes could be divided in eubacteria and archaebacteria.

However, subsequently, it was shown that this group archaea is distinct from bacteria and eukaryotes (Table). The living cells are, therefore, now divided into the following three domains: bacteria, archaea and eukarya.

Such a classification in three domains has been proved more conclusively in the year 1996, when the genome of an archaeon, namely Methanococcus jannaschii was fully sequenced (nucleotide sequence fully determined) and compared with sequences of the genomes of bacteria and eukaryotes.

{During 1995-2000, nucleotide sequences of complete genomes of ~ 45 other organisms were worked out. These organisms largely involved prokaryotes, but also included the following four eukaryotes: budding yeast (Saccharomyces cerevisiae), a nematode (Coenorhabditis elegans), fruitfly (Drosophila melanogaster) and a weed of mustard family (Arabidopsis thaliana). Genomes of about 300 other organisms were also being sequenced at the end of the year 2000}.

A Comparison of Prokaryotic Organisms (bacteria and cyanobacteria) and Eukaryotic Organisms (protists, fungi, plants and animals)

Feature	*Prokaryotes*	*Eukaryotes*
1. Cell size and cell organisation	1-10 μ m, unicellular (many cell types)	5-100 μ m; multicellular
2. Organelles	Few or none	Nucleus, mitochondria, chloroplasts, endoplasmic reticulum, golgi apparatus, etc.
3. DNA	Circular (or linear) DNA organised in a nucleoid	Linear DNA molecules organised in chromosomes bounded in a nucleus
4. Synthesis of RNA and proteins	RNA and proteins synthesized in same compartment	RNA synthesized and processed in the nucleus; proteins synthesized in the cytoplasm
5. Cytoskeleton	Absent	Present
6. Spindle apparatus in cell division	Absent; replicated DNA pulled by attachment to plasma membrane	Present; chromosomes pulled by spindle apparatus
7. Metabolism	Anaerobic/aerobic	Aerobic

In Archaea, the Distribution of Eukaryotic, Prokaryotic and Novel Unique Genes

Eukaryotic genes	*Prokaryotic genes*	*Novel unique genes*
1. DNA replication	1. Transport of inorganic ions (*e.g.*, Na^+, K^+) across	1. Only one DNA polymerase the cell
2. Transcription	2. Cell surface structure	2. Several tRNA aminoacyl synthetase enzymes missing
3. Translation		3. Numerous inteins (18 in all) are known that are inserted intoproteins and then removed
4. Histone genes.		

During an expedition to deep sea, M. jannaschii was

discovered in 1982 from a hot spot, three kilometers beneath the pacific ocean and was found to be a methane producing organism. It was named Methanococcus jannaschii after Holger

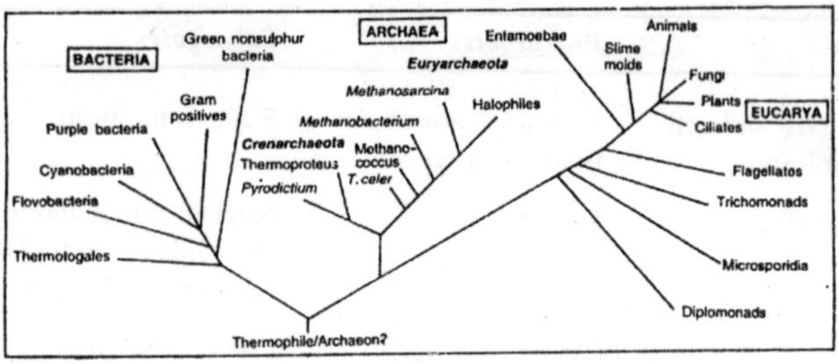

Evolution of three major life forms (prokarya, archaea and eukarya) from a common ancestor (a thermophile).

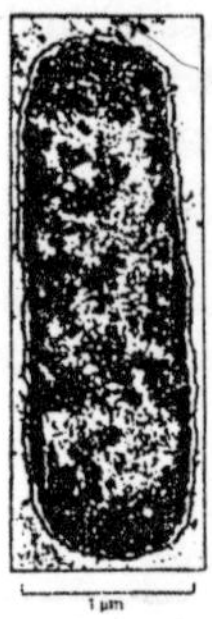

A bacterial cell showing details of internal structure.

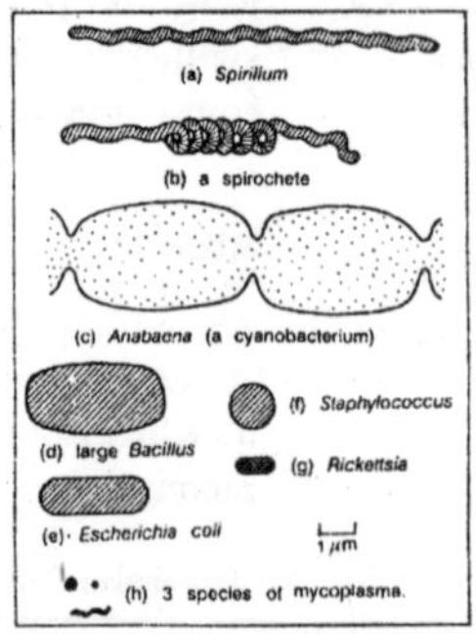

Some prokaryotic cells drawn to scale (redrawn from Alberts *et al.*; *Molecular Biology of the Cell*, 1994).

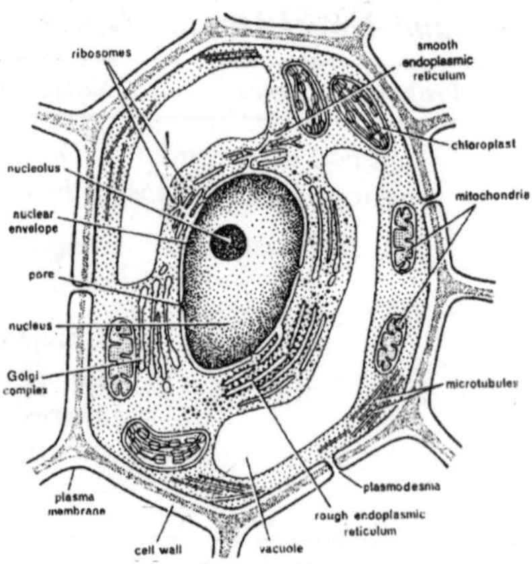

Structure of a plant cell.

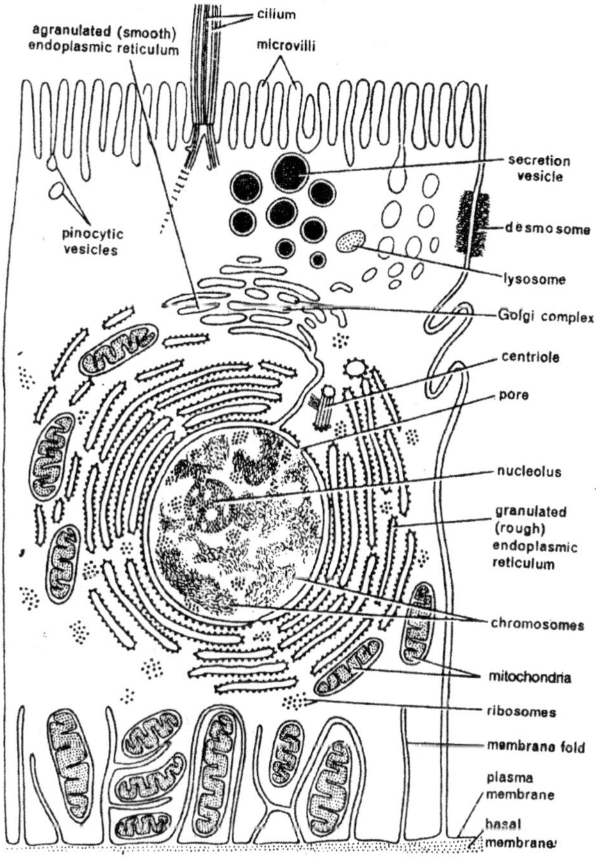

Structure of an animal cell.

Jannasch, the expedition leader. Following are some of the novel features of this archaeon forcing biologists to place it in a new domain archaea, distinct from bacteria and eukarya. (i) 56 per cent of the archaeon's genes are new to science; (ii) it lives at temperatures ranging from 48°C to 94°C and at pressures of more than 200 atmospheres (some archaea grow at salt concentrations up to 10 times higher than that of sea water); oxygen kills it; it is an autotroph utilising carbon dioxide, nitrogen and hydrogen; it produces methane and thus is a methanogen; (iii) there are archaeon's genes that resemble those of bacteria, others that resemble eukaryotes and still others that are completely new to science.

It has also been shown that the archaeal system is more like a eukaryotic system. In fact scientists now believe that the common ancestor of all modern living creatures was a thermophile (heat loving), which branched off more than 3.6 billion years ago into three major life forms, prokaryotes (bacteria), archaea and eukarya (Fig.).

The structure of a bacterial cell (prokaryote) is shown in Figure. The variation in the size of some prokaryotic cells is shown in Figure. The structures of eukaryotic plant and animal cells are respectively shown in Figures.

Eukaryotic Cells are Organised into Compartments: Earlier in the history of cytology, the cytologists used to divide a eukaryotic cell into two important compartments, (i) the nucleus and (ii) the cytoplasm. In later years with the development of electron microscope, it became possible to study the cytoplasm as well as the nucleus in greater details. As a result, various kinds of inclusions have been discovered to be present outside the nucleus in the cytoplasm. These inclusions are known as cell organelles.

The discovery of these various kinds of cell organelles made the definition of the term cytoplasm more and more difficult. The more important cell organelles are (i) nucleus, which controls all the activities of the cell, (ii) plastids, which are involved in the formation and storage of carbohydrates, (iii) mitochondria, which are the power houses of the cell and supply all energy needed for the maintenance of life, (iv) endoplasmic reticulum, which performs an active role in protein synthesis and transport, (v) ribosomes which are the sites of protein synthesis, (vi) endosomes, (vii) lysosomes, which are primarily rich in enzymes and are lytic in nature, (viii) golgi bodies which are secretory in nature and

(ix) peroxisomes and hydrogenosomes, (x) centrosome, which takes part in organisation and function of spindle apparatus.

The natural question, therefore, can be asked whether the cytoplasm should be something devoid of all these cell organelles or should it include all these organelles except the nucleus. It has been suggested by some workers, that it would be convenient to use the term cytoplasm for the matrix or the fluid present outside the nucleus excluding mitochondria and plastids.

According to another terminology, the general area of the cell excluding all membrane bound compartments, is described as cytosol. Other closed compartments are called cell organelles (as described above). Among these cell organelles, mitochondria and plastids have their own self-replicating machinery like the nucleus and are, therefore, independent. Moreover, although previously it was believed that DNA (the sole genetic material) is located only in the nucleus, now there is definite evidence that DNA is found in plastids and mitochondria also. There is also evidence that the function of plastid DNA and mitochondrial DNA is similar to that of nuclear DNA.

Therefore, the cell structure, whose ground plan for a plant cell is given in Figure and that for an animal cell is given in Figure, will be discussed in the following heads; (i) extracellular matrix (ECM) and cell wall, (ii) cell membrane, (iii) nucleus, (iv) mitochondria, (v) plastids, (vi) ER, ribosomes, endosomes and lysosomes, peroxisomes and hydrogenosomes, centrosomes, (vii) cytoskeleton, etc.

3

Chemical Aspects

Cells are actually regarded as macromolecular assemblies. These macromolecules, making 30 per cent of the cell's mass (70 per cent of cell's mass is water), include proteins, nucleic acids and polysaccharides. Though lipids are also large molecules, they are not large enough to be classified as macromolecules. Among the classes of macromolecules, proteins and nucleic acids are very large molecules, responsible for conveying genetic information. While nucleic acids carry the genetic information from one cell generation to another, proteins provide a means of expressing this genetic information.

Polysaccharides are also big enough to be classified as macromolecules, but they do not have the complexity of proteins and nucleic acids to carry-or express the information. Of the three classes of macromolecules, proteins have the highest of diversity, nucleic acids have some diversity and polysaccharides have the lowest level of diversity.

These macromolecules are polymers of small micromolecules (proteins are polymers of amino acids, nucleic acids are polymers of nucleotides and polysaccharides are polymers of monosaccharide sugar molecules). Each macromolecule has (i) a backbone consisting of a regularly repeating series of bonds and (ii) side groups branching out from the backbone and providing characteristic diversity. The bonds connecting the monomers and the side groups known in the above three macromolecules are presented in Table and Figure.

Bonds in the Backbone and the Side Groups of Biological Macromolecules

Macromolecule backbone side	*Nature of groups (*)*	*Nature of*
1. Proteins	Peptide	Amino acids (20)
2. Nucleic acids	Sugar-phosphate bond (phospho-diester bond)	Nitrogenous bases (4)
3. Polysaccharides	Glycosidic bond	Hydroxyl group or substituent (-)

(*) figures in parentheses are number of types in each case.

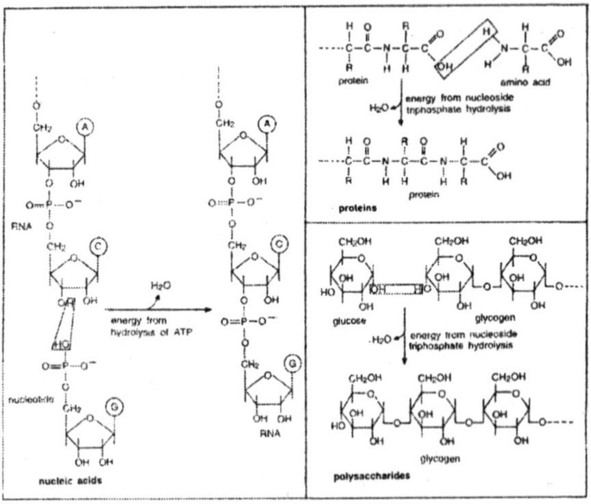

Derivation of three types of macromolecules (polymers) from their monomers due to formation of three kinds of bonds.

Covalent and Weak Non-Covalent Bonds in Macro-molecules: The structure of macromolecules is achieved and maintained with the help of strong covalent bonds and some weak non-covalent bonds. Therefore it is necessary to understand the nature of these bonds, before we discuss the structure of macromolecules.

The monomers in a macromolecular chain (a polymer) are held together by covalent bonds, which are formed between atoms due to sharing of one or more electrons (in a single bond, one electron from each atom is shared; in a double bond a total of four electrons are shared). Atoms joined by two or more covalent bonds can not rotate freely about the bond axis and this influences three-dimensional shape of many macromolecules. These covalent bonds are strong enough (particularly in water) to preserve the sequence of subunits for a long time (Table); their formation may need enzymes, and their strength is not affected by the environment.

Covalent Bonds and Non-covalent Bonds Differ in Strength

Type of bond	*Length of bond (nm)*	*Strength of bond (kcal/mole) (energy required to break a bond)*	
		in vacuum	*in water*
1. Covalnet	0.15	90	90
2. Ionic	0.25	80	3
3. Hydrogen	0.30	4	1
4. Van der Waals (per atom)	0.35	1.0	0.1
5. Hydrophobic	—	3	0.5

The weak bonds, on the other hand, are formed between different parts of the same macromolecule or between different macromolecules. Their formation, which does not need any enzymes, is strongly influenced by the aqueous environment.

Thus these weak bonds determine not only the secondary and tertiary structures of these macromolecules, but also determine their distribution and arrangement within a cell. These weak bonds thus are indispensable for the very existence of the cell. In view of this, an understanding of these weak interactions is necessary to understand the structure and function of macromolecules.

Spontaneous formation of a bond always involves release of energy, and breaking of this bond will similarly consume energy; the stronger the bond greater the amount of energy released. In a cell, bonds are regularly formed and broken, so that at an equilibrium the number of bonds formed is equal to the number of bonds broken. The proportion of bonded molecules is described by the following formula, where Keq is the equilibrium constant.

$$A + B \rightarrow AB + \text{energy}$$

$$K_{eq} = \frac{\text{Conc. of AB}}{\text{Conc. of A} \times \text{Conc. of B}}$$

At this equilibrium, the change in free energy is zero ($\Delta G=0$) and the amount of this free energy is minimum. (Free energy is the energy that has the ability to do work).

Four types of non-covalent bonds that occur in macromolecules include (i) ionic bonds, (ii) hydrogen bonds, (iii) Van der Waals forces, (iv) hydrophobic interactions.

Ionic Interactions

Ionic interactions occur between oppositely charged groups (ions). These interactions may occur between fully charged groups (ionic bonds) or between partially charged groups. The force of attraction between the charges q^+andq^- is defined by Coulomb's law, which says that force = $(q^+q^-)/r^2 D$ (where D= dielectric constant, which is 1 for vacuum and 80 for water; r= distance of separation). In the absence of water, in solids these forces are very strong as in salt (NaCl) or marble.

In NaCl, the force between Na^+ and Cl^- has a strength comparable to covalent bond. However in solution, water molecules interact with charged group in such a way that water shields the charge, thus weakening the ionic bond. In a protein, acidic and basic amino acids may also interact forming ionic bonds; similarly a protein molecule having a charged group may interact with another protein molecule (protein-protein interaction) or other target molecule like nucleic acid (protein-nucleic acid interaction) having an opposite charge. Another example of ionic interactions is that between an enzyme and its substrate.

Hydrogen Bonds

Hydrogen bonds are weak electrostatic bonds, in which a hydrogen atom is shared between two other atoms, both electronegative, as between O and N or between O and O in the following examples.

>C = O - - - - - - - - - - - - - H-N-

hydrogen bond convalent bond

(—0.2nm) (-0.1 nm)

>C = O - - - - - - - - - - - - - H-O-

In proteins, hydrogens bonds are formed between NH and CO groups of the peptide backbone. Hydrogen bonds may also involve side groups in a protein chain. The commonest example of hydrogen bonds is the bonds between different molecules of liquid water (Fig.) or between water molecules and other molecules. Hydrogen bonds also occur between amino acids in a polypeptide chain or between hydroxyl groups of two different molecules (Fig.).

Many organic molecules also possess ionic groups with charges which are neutralised by nearby, oppositely charged groups within these organic molecules or by inorganic ions

(Na^+ , K^+, Mg^{++}, Cl^-, SO_4^+). But, directional bonds are formed, if oppositely charged groups can form hydrogen bonds (*e.g.* COO^- and NH_3^+ may be held together by hydrogen bonds; when such hydrogen bonds are formed between ionic groups, ionic bonds are hydrogen bonds; Fig.).

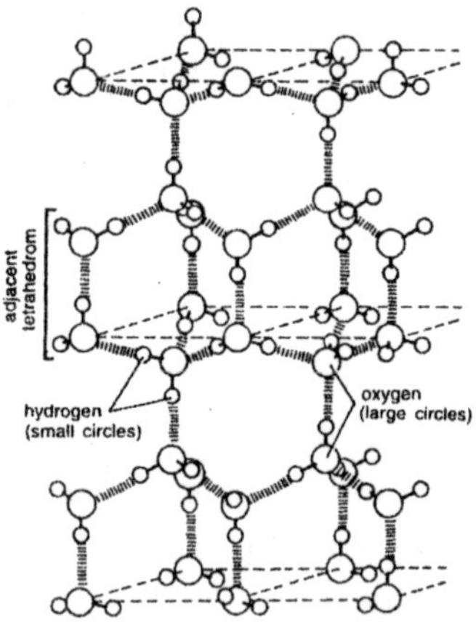

Formation of hydrogen bond between different molecules of water.

Van der Waals bonding

Van der Waals bonding results due to nonspecific attractive force between atoms which come close to each other. In this case there are no permanent charges associated with participating groups, but there are fluctuating charges induced due to nearness of molecules. Therefore these bonds occur among nonpolar as well as polar molecules and their strength depends on the distance between interacting groups (Fig.). If these atoms are brought very close to each other, they will very strongly repel each other and this Van der Waals repulsion plays a major role in maintaining the conformation of biological molecules. However, at a particular distance between atoms (which is specific for each type of atom), attraction and repulsion forces balance each other (Fig.). This distance is called Van der Waals radius (Table). Interaction between antigen and antibody may also be due to such Van der Waals forces.

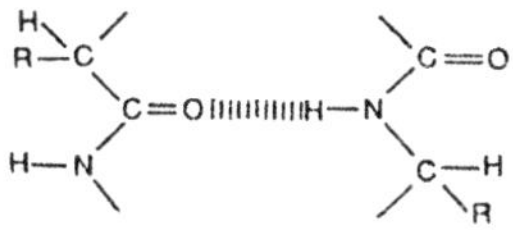

(a) hydrogen bond between peptide groups

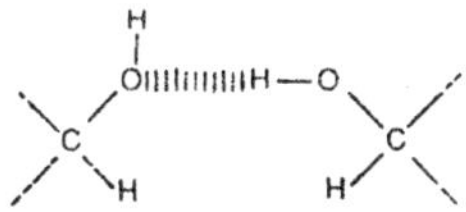

(b) hydrogen bond between two hydroxyl groups

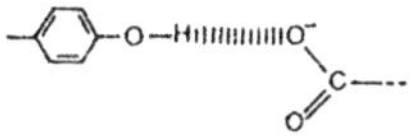

(c) hydrogen bond between a charged carboxyl group and the hydroxyl group of tyrosine

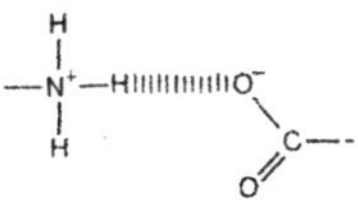

(d) hydrogen bond between a charged amino group and a charged carboxyl group

Formation of hydrogen bonds (a) between amino acids in a polypeptide,
(b) between two hydroxyl groups,
(c) between a carboxyl group and a hydroxyl group and
(d) between amino group and a carboxyl group

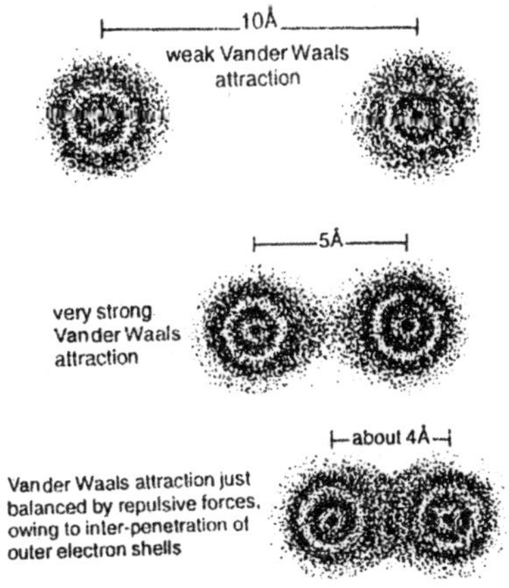

Van der Waals bonds, showing dependence of their strength on the distance between interacting groups.

Van der Waals Radii of Atoms in Biological Molecules

Atom	*Van der Waal's Radius*	*Atom*	*Van der Waal's Radius*
H	1.2 Å	P	1.90 Å
N	1.5 Å	S	1.85 Å
O	1.4 Å	C	2.00 Å

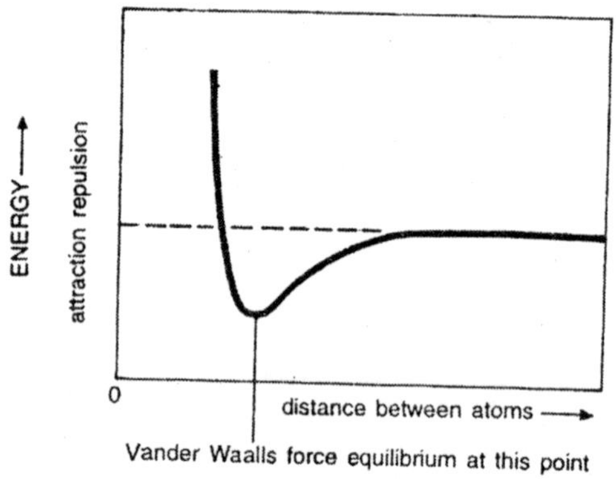

Relationship between Van der Waals force (attraction/repulsion) and the distance between atoms.

Hydrophobic Bonds

Hydrophobic bonds result not due to any attraction, but only due to a tendency of water to exclude or repel the nonpolar groups. In view of this the term bond is a misnomer, although it serves a useful purpose by emphasising that the molecules arrange to avoid contact with water molecules. These so called hydrophobic bonds help not only in stabilisation of proteins or their complexes with other molecules, but also in partitioning of proteins into membranes.

Various Acids

Nucleic acids are the most important macromolecules in the cells of all organisms. In the beginning of the 20th century it was shown that chromosomes (consisting mainly of nucleic acids and proteins) within a cell carry the hereditary factors. However, for several decades, we did not know whether nucleic acids or proteins are the carriers of genetic information. In 1940's and 1950's, several experiments demonstrated that nucleic acids are the genetic material within the cells. Some of these experiments will be briefly discussed before we discuss the structure of these macromolecules.

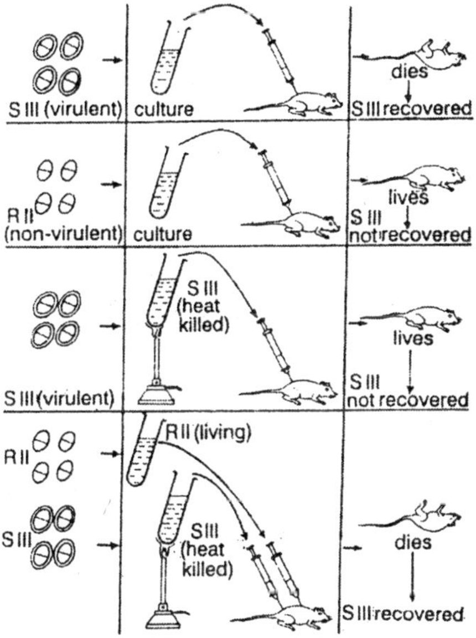

Griffith's experiment demosntrating transformation in pneumococcus.

Nucleic Acids as Genetic Material

Chromosomes mainly consist of nucleoproteins having two components, nucleic acids and proteins. One of these should obviously constitute the genetic material.

Transformation Experiments: Transformation experiments were initially conducted by F. Griffith in 1928. He injected a mixture of two strains of pneumococcus (Diplococcus pneumoniae) into mice. One of these two strains, SIII was virulent and the other strain RII was non virulent (causing no infection). Heat killed virulent strain SIII, when injected individually did not cause death, showing that infectivity after heat killing is lost. The mice injected with a mixture of RII (living) and SIII (heat killed) died and virulent pneumococci could be isolated from these mice (Fig.). This phenomenon was described as transformation.

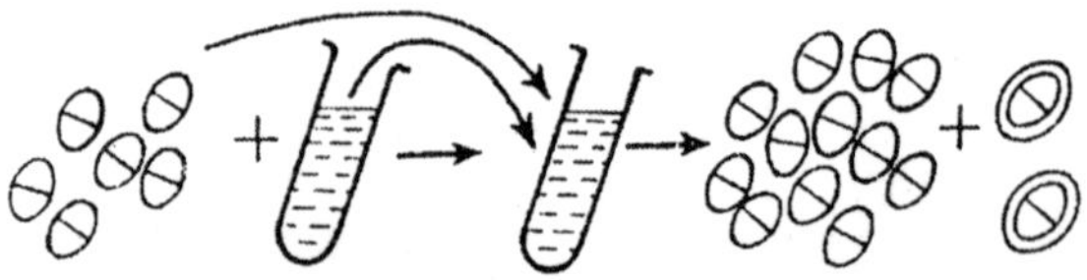

Transformation experiment of Avery et. al., (1944).

O.T. Avery, C.M. Macleod and M. McCarthy repeated Griffith's experiments in an in vitro system in order to identify the transforming substance responsible for converting non-virulent into virulent type and reported their results in 1944. Virulence in pneumococcus depends on a polysaccharide capsule which is present in virulent strain SIII and is absent in non- virulent strain RII.

The cells of non-capsulated type (RII) were treated with an extract of DNA from capsulated strain SIII. A few cells of SIII type could be isolated from the mixture (Fig.). This phenomenon of transferring characters of one strain to another by using a DNA extract of the former is called transformation. When the extract was treated with DNAase (an enzyme which destroys DNA) this transforming ability was lost. Proteases (enzymes which destroy proteins) did not affect the transforming ability. These experiments thus indicated that DNA and not the proteins is the genetic material.

Experiments with bacteriophage (T2) infection. The fact that DNA is the genetic material could also be demostrated with the help of infecting bacteria by bacteriophage known as T2. This phage consists of proteins and DNA. The complex structure of a T2 phage particle is shown is Figures. It consists of a head and a tail. The head consists of protein coat and DNA. The tail similarly consists of tail core, tail sheath and tail fibres. The phage attaches to the host bacterium with the help of tail fibres. After infection, multiplication of phage occurs and a large number of progeny phages, genetically similar to the infecting phage are produced.

In 1952, A.D. Hershey and M.J. Chase reported results of experiments which demonstrated that only DNA of the phage enters host cells and that this DNA carries all the genetic information necessary for assembly of new phage progeny.

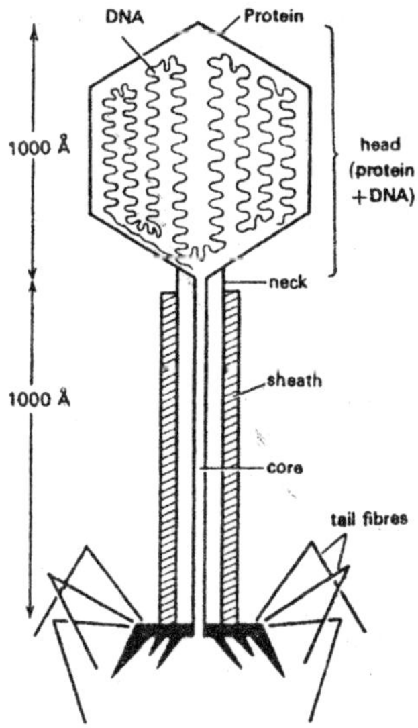

Structure of T2 Bacteriophage.

In these experiments, phage DNA was made radioactive by growing infected bacteria on a medium containing $^{32}PO_4$. Since phage proteins do not contain phosphorus, only DNA would be labelled. Similarly, phage proteins were labelled with the help of $^{35}SO_4$. Since DNA does not contain sulphur, only protein would be labelled with ^{35}S. Such differential labelling would enable one to distinguish between DNA and proteins of the phage without performing any chemical tests. Hershey and Chase then allowed both kinds of labelled phage particles to infect bacteria. The infected· bacteria were immediately agitated in a waring blender. After shaking, only radioactive ^{32}P was found associated with bacterial cells and ^{35}S was found only in surrounding medium and not in bacterial cells. When phage progeny was studied for radioactivity in this experiment,, it was found that the phage, progeny carried label only with ^{32}P. The progeny was not labelled with ^{35}S. This experiment is diagrammatically represented in Figure and clearly indicated that only DNA and not protein enters the bacterial cells. The protein coat is left outside.

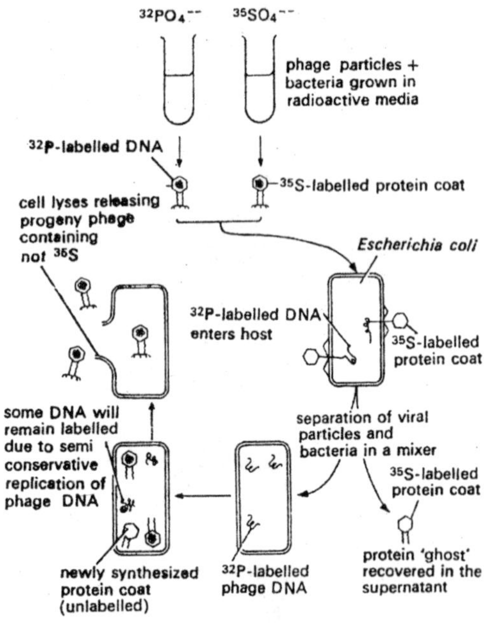

Experiment of Hershey and Chase, where DNA of bacteriophage is labelled with ^{32}p and the protein is labelled with ^{35}S.

This DNA entering the host cell carries all the genetic information, for synthesis of new phage particles. Indirectly, this experiment conducted by Hershey and Chase proved that DNA is the sole genetic material in DNA bacteriophages. A.D. Hershey shared with M. Dellbruck and S.E. Luria, the Nobel Prize in Medicine/ Physiology for 1969.

Experiments with tobacco mosaic virus (TMV). With the help of transformation experiment and bacteriophage infection discussed above, it was shown that DNA is the genetic material. The first evidence that RNA also has the capacity to carry genetic information came from experiments conducted with tobacco mosaic virus (TMV). This virus does not contain any DNA, and is composed of RNA (6%) surrounded by a hollow cylinder of protein subunits. The experiments conducted by H. Fraenkel-Conrat in California showing that RNA is the genetic material in this virus.

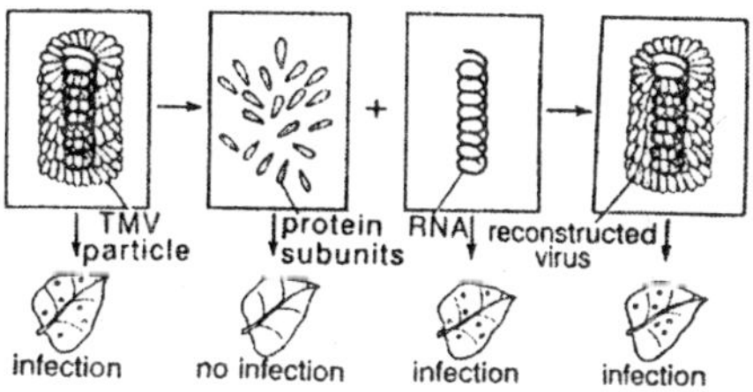

Experiment of Fraenkel-Conrat on TMV showing that RNA and not the protein can cause infection.

Techniques were first developed for separating TMV particles into RNA and proteins. Later by using RNA and proteins separately in tests for infectivity, it could be shown that RNA alone was able to cause infection. Such a property was not found in the protein fraction (Fig.). It was also possible to synthesize chimeric virus particles using RNA from one strain and protein from another strain. Such chimeras had serological properties of those strains from which protein was derived, but in other properties, it resembled the other strain from which RNA was used.

In one experiment, two viruses used were tobacco mosaic virus (TMV) and Holmes rib-grass virus (HRV). The latter was isolated from Plantago lanceolata and therefore, is also known as Plantago strain. Proteins of these two viruses differ in having different frequencies and sequences of amino acids. Also these viruses give different symptoms. On leaves of a particular virus gives progeny, which resembles the virus from which RNA was derived.

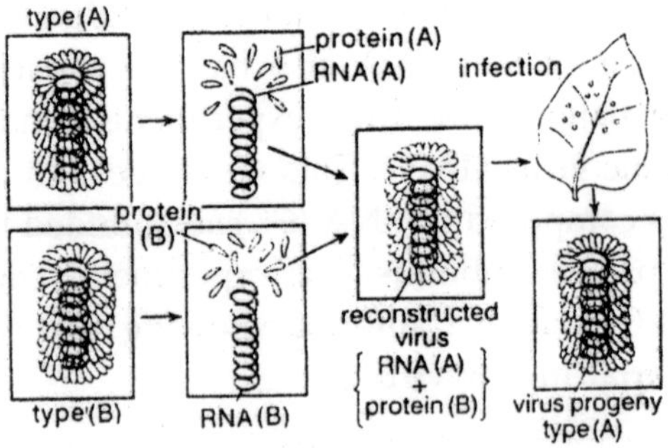

Reconstruction of virus, showing that reconstructed

Variety of tobacco, while TMV produces mottling of leaves, HRV produces distinct ring patterns. Reciprocal chimeras using RNA of one strain and protein of the other strain could be obtained. It was found that when these chimeras were used for infection, the progeny had proteins which corresponded to the virus from which RNA of the infecting virus particles was derived. This proved that specificity of virus proteins was determined by RNA alone and the proteins carried no information. Results of these experiments are diagrammatically represented in Figure.

Subsequently, after the demonstration of genetic nature of RNA in TMV, RNA was found in a number of bacteriophages. Therefore, it may be concluded that nucleic acids in general, RNA as well as DNA, carry genetic information. However, DNA perhaps always functions as genetic material ; but RNA in majority of cases is non-genetic; only in specific systems where DNA is absent, it functions as genetic material. In recent years, RNA has been shown to functions as enzymes (ribozymes) also. This aspect of RNA led to award of Nobel Prize in chemistry in 1989 (T. Cech and S. Altman). 'Prions' have also been described in recent years as 'proteinaceous infectious particles' which is an example of 'protein conformation based inheritance'. Nobel Prize for 1997 was awarded to Stanley B. Prusiner for the discovery of 'prions'.

Structure of Nucleic Acids (Polynucleotides)

Nucleic acid molecule is a long chain polymer (polynucleotide) composed of monomeric units, called nucleotides. These nucleotide monomer units are joined by the formation of phosphodiester bonds (a diester bond is one which involves two ester bonds). A phosphodiester bond will be formed between any two adjacent nucleotides.

A polynucleotide chain (Fig.) would have a direction so that, if it starts from C^3 it would end in C^5 and if it starts from C^5 it would end in C^3. Normally, therefore, whether we are referring to a mononucleotide or else to a polynucleotide we should indicate the groups present at C^3 end and at C^5 end.

It could be either a phosphate group or a hydroxyl group. For instance, 5'pApT.OH3'dinucleotide would mean that it is a polynucleotide with only two nucleotide units acid has phosphate group at the 5 end and a hydroxyl group at the 3' end.

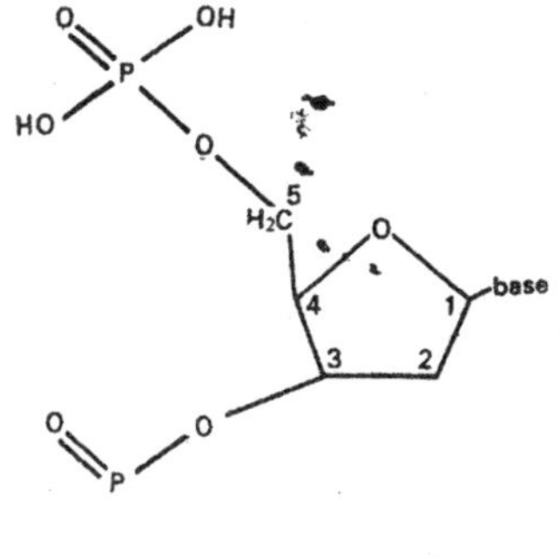

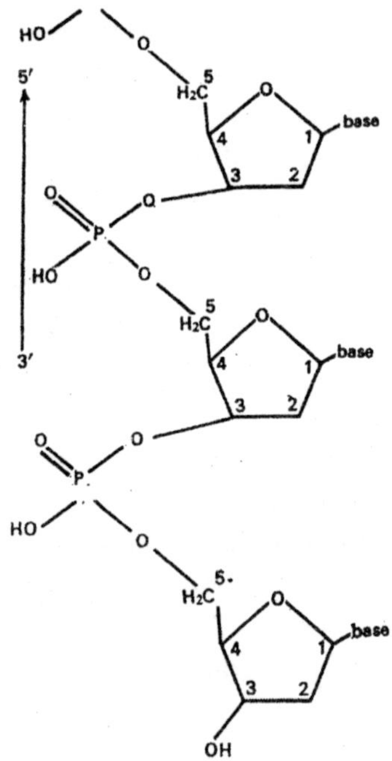

A polynucleotide chain showing phosphodiester bonds.

A short hand notation of a polynucleotide (or oligonucleotide) with a constitution 5'AGCT3' or 5'pApGpCpT-OH3' is shown is Figure. This is a very convenient method to write nucleotide sequences with 5' terminus on the left and 3' terminus or the right side. In this notation the vertical lines represent the pentose sugars, each with 5 carbon atoms.

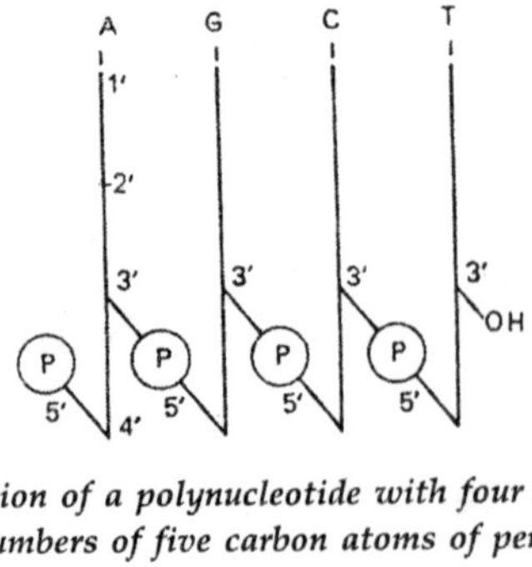

A short-hand notation of a polynucleotide with four nucleotides (1 'to 5' represent numbers of five carbon atoms of pentose sugar).

Deoxyribonucleic acid (DNA). J.D. Watson and F.H.C. Crick showed in 1953 that DNA has a double helical structure with two polynucleotide chains connected by hydrogen bonds and running in opposite directions. When DNA samples are analysed from different organs of body of the same individual or from different individuals belonging to the same species, no differences in the relative composition of different bases were observed. The following generalisations could also be made: (i) Number of adenine molecules always equalled number of thymine molecules, (ii) Number of cytosine molecules always equalled number of guanine molecules, (iii) Number of adenine molecules did not necessarily equal that of guanine and similar relationship was observed between cytosine and thymine.

Although A = T and C = G, there is no restriction on the ratio (A + T)/(C + G); nor is there any restriction on sequence of bases in one polynucleotide chain. But, since A is always linked to T and C to G as determined from the above evidences, sequence of bases in one polynucleotide should determine the sequence of bases in the other polynucleotide of the double helix.

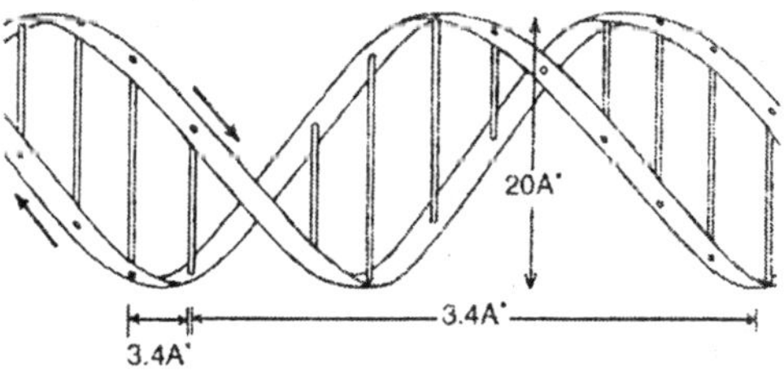

A double helix model of DNA as proposed by Watson and Crick.

Besides chemical analysis, DNA was also studied by X-ray crystallography by M.H.F. Wilkins and his associates. Such studies demonstrated that DNA was a helical structure with a diameter of 20 Å and a pitch (one round) of about 34 Å. On the basis of these studies of chemical analysis and X-ray crystallography, following features of the DNA molecule are now known: (i) DNA consists of a double helix, in which two poly-nucleotide chains are coiled about the same axis in such a fashion that they can separate from one another only be uncoiling and that lateral separation would not be possible, (ii) Bases are set in a plane at right angle to the long axis, (iii) Two polynucleotide chains' which run in opposite directions, have complementary base sequences, since adenine is linked to thymine and cytosine to guanine. (iv) Distance between two base pairs is 3.4 A° and there are 10 base pairs in each turn.

Choice of base pairing is understandable because of a constant diameter of 20 A° in the molecule; two purines would need too much space and two pyrimidines would occupy too little space to pair. When a pyrimidine always pairs with a purine, space could remain constant. The pattern of coiling of two polynucleotide chains is shown in Figure .

Alternative Forms of DNA Double Helices: The well known structure of DNA described above pertains to DNA structure, described by Watson and Crick (1953). Helical coiling of this DNA is assumed to be right handed and this form of DNA has been called B-form. It has been shown that DNA may also exist in other alternative forms of double helical structures.

These alternative forms differ in features like (i) number of residues per turn ('n') or (ii) the spacing of residues along the helical axis ('h'). The existence of DNA as a double helix has also been confirmed by experiments used to measure the number of base pairs per turn and it has been shown that this is 10.4 instead of 10.0 shown in classical B-form. This will lead to modification of the twist angle (rotation) between two base pairs from 36° to 34.6° (360°/10.4).

This figure of 10.4 base pairs per turn is an average and according to conditions, this may shift in either direction. It is thus obvious that there may be several families of structures of DNA, each of a characteristic type showing variation in the values of 'n' and 'h' described above. Three structural forms, namely A, B and C are known for a long time and transitions between them can occur, General characteristics of these" three forms are given in Table.

Several forms of DNA Double Helical Structures

Helix type	*Conditions*	*Base pairs per turn*	*Rotation per bp*	*Vertical rise per bp (h)*	*Helical diameter*
A	75% rel. humidity; Na^+ K^+, Cs^+ ions	11	+32.7° (right handed)	2.3 Å	25.5 Å
B	92% rel. humidity; low ionic strength	10	+36.0° (right handed)	3.4 Å	23.7 Å
C	66% rel. humidity; Li^+ ions	9.33	+38.6° right handed)	3.3 Å	23.7 Å
Z	Very high salt concentration	12	-30.0° (left handed)	5.7 Å	18.4 Å

The B-form is found at a very high (92%) relative humidity and low ionic strength. Similarly, A-form is found at 75 per cent relative humidity in the presence of Na^+ K^+, or Cs^+ ions and C-form is found at 60 per cent relative humidity in the presence of Li^+ (Lithium) ions. These three forms are assumed to be found in all DNAs. There are still other forms called D-form and E-form found rarely as extreme variants with only 8 and 7½ base pairs per turn respectively. These are found only in some DNA molecules lacking guanine. In contrast A, B, and C are found in all DNA molecules irrespective of DNA sequence. As shown in Table, B DNA is not the only right handed DNA. Similarly, it has been shown that B DNA is not always right handed. B DNA can also be left handed.

Z-DNA, a left handed DNA form: Another form of DNA has been obtained artificially by synthesizing $d(C\text{-}G)_3$ molecules which were isolated as crystals. This form of DNA has also been detected in living cells using specific antibodies raised against it. Because this form of DNA follows a zig-zag course, it has been called Z-DNA. It resembles the B form in many respects and differs from it in many other respects (Table). The differences and similarities are described below:

Resemblances Between z-DNA and B-DNA: (i) Both are double helical, (ii) Two strands of double helix are antiparallel in both DNAs. (iii) Both forms exhibit A=T and G=C pairing.

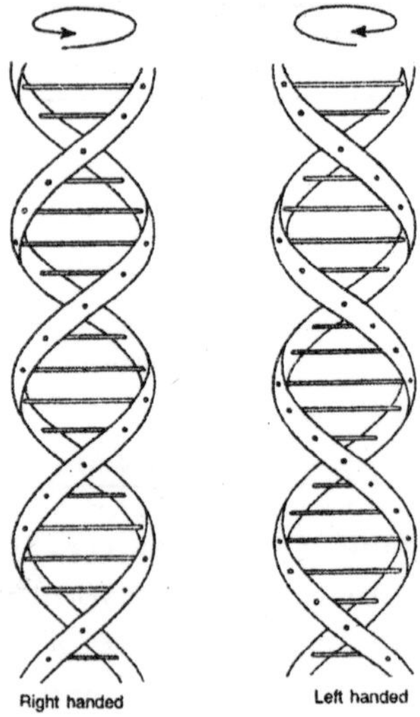

Two helicals, one showing right handed sense as found in B-DNA and the other showing left handed sense as found in Z- DNA.

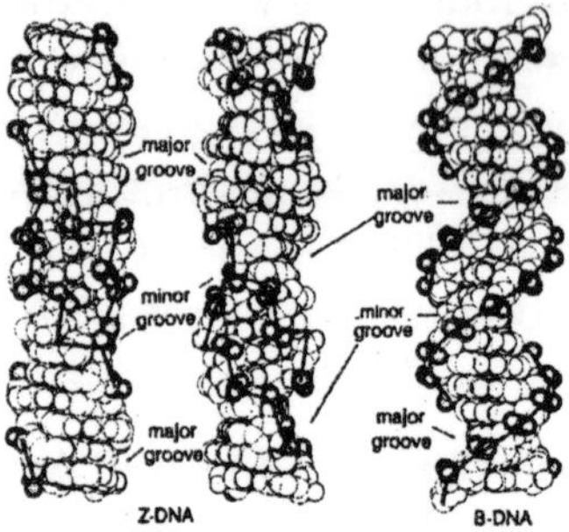

Side views of Z-DNA and B-DNA. Two views of Z-DNA are 30° apart. Irregularity of backbone in Z-DNA is shown by heavy lines showing the path of phosphate residues, which is quite regular and smooth in B-DNA (redrawn from Nature, Vol. 282, 1979).

Differences between z-DNA and B-DNA (i) Z-DNA has left-handed helical sense as against right handed helical sense of B-DNA (Fig.). (ii) Due to a different arrangement of molecules within Z-DNA polymer, phosphate backbone follows a zig-zag course, while in B- DNA it is regular (Fig.). (iii) In Z-DNA, sugar residues of a polynucleotide chain have alternating orientation (Fig.) so that repeating unit is a dinucleotide as against B-DNA where repeating unit is a mononucleotide and the orientation of sugar molecules is not alternating, (iv) In Z-DNA, one complete helix, *i.e.*, a twist through 360°, has twelve base pairs or six repeating dinucleotide units (12 base pairs), while in B-DNA, one complete helix has only ten base pairs or ten repeating units, (v) Because twelve base pairs are accommodated in one helix in Z-DNA, as against ten in B-DNA, the angle of twist per repeating unit (dinucleotide) is 60° as against 36° in B-DNA. (vi) One complete helix is 45 Å in Z-DNA, while it is 34 Å in B- DNA. (vii) Since bases get more length to spread out in Z-DNA and since the angle of tilt is 60°, they are closer to the axis and hence the diameter of Z-DNA molecule is 18 Å, whereas it is 20 Å in B-DNA.

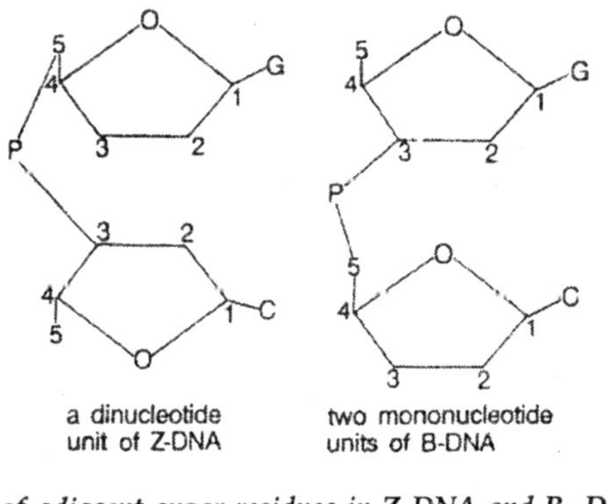

Orientation of adjacent sugar residues in Z-DNA and B- DNA showing opposite orientations in Z-DNA and same orientation in B-DNA. This results in dinucleotide units in Z-DNA as against mononucleotide units in B-DNA.

In addition to the above, other differences include (i) differences in glycosidic torsion angle, which is anti in B-DNA and syn in Z-DNA for deoxyguanosine and (ii) differences in sugar pucker which is C_2' endo for B-DNA and C_3' endo for Z-DNA in deoxyguanosine.

The situation is reverse for deoxycytidine. These differences are summarised in Table.

Comparison of Helices of B-DNA and Z-DNA (from Nature, 282, 1979).

	B-DNA	*Z-DNA*
1. Helix sense	Right handed	Left handed
2. Residues per turn	10	12 (6 dimers)
3. Diameter	-20 Å	-18 Å
4. Rise per residue	3.4 Å	3.75 Å
5. Helix pitch	34 Å	45 Å
6. Base pair tilt	16°	7°
7. Rotation per residue	36°	60* (per dimer)
8. Glycoside torsion angle,		
deoxyguanosine	Anti	% Syn
deoxycytidine	Anti	Anti
9. Sugar pucker,		
deoxyguanoise	C_2' endo	C_3' endo
deoxycytidine	C_3' endo	C_2' endo
10. Distance of P from axis,		
dGpC	9.0 Å	8.0 Å
dCpG	9.0 Å	6.9 Å

In vivo existence and role of Z-DNA? A few years ago, it was suggested that Z-DNA may be transient configuration of—DNA in living cells and may thus play a role in (i) regulation of gene activity and/or in (ii) genetic recombination. Earlier the role of Z-DNA in regulation of gene activity was suggested, since Z-DNA specific antibodies could bind specifically to interband regions of salivary gland chromosomes and not to active banded regions. This suggested that Z-DNA conformation renders the DNA inactive. These observations were later shown to be an artefact of chromosome fixation. However, sequences capable of forming Z-DNA are believed to play a role in recombination or rearrangement of DNA (*e.g.* immunoglobulin genes).

RL Model by Sasizekharan: During 1976-80, V. Sasizekharan and his coworkers, of Indian Institute of Science, Bangalore, emphasised that the right handed form (R) of double helical B-DNA can not easily explain the unwinding of the duplex due to topological difficulties. They suggested that right handed (R) and left handed (L) double helices are equally likely and therefore proposed a new RL model. In this model a B-DNA structure with alternating right handed and left handed segments of approximately five base pairs, in a repeat of ten base pairs, was proposed. This model provides for conformational flexibility. The essential differences between the right handed (R) double helix of Watson and Crick and the RL model of Sasizekharan are given in Table. There is strong experimental evidence available in favour of RL model, although one does not know the possible maximum continuous lengths of right handed and left handed segments of DNA.

Supercoils in Closed DNA: The double helix structure of DNA represents a linear DNA molecule, but DNA in vivo often has a closed structure without any free ends.

A Comparison between Right Handed (R) and RL Models

Properties	*Watson and Crick's 'R' model*	*Sasizekharan's 'RL' model*
1. Helix sense	Right handed throughout	Alternating right and left handed segments
2. Rotation/10 bp	360°	0° to 36° (ideally 0')
3. Conformational flexibility	No	Yes

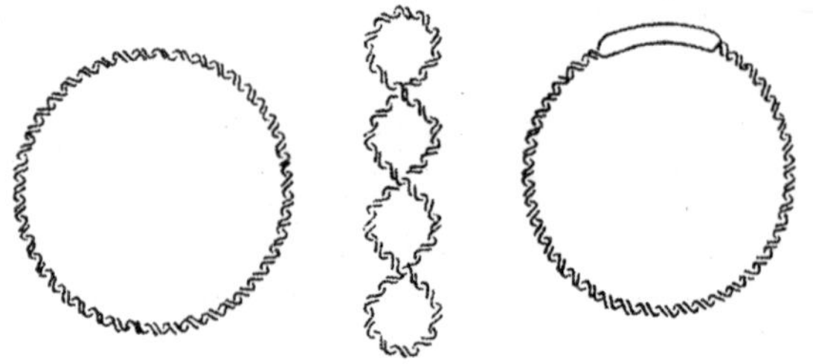

Supercoiling of DNA leading to a twisted duplex, which may be undone by strand separation in a region.

In bacteria and viruses, DNA is often circular. In eukaryotes also, large loops of DNA are found in such a way that each loop represents part of a circle. This organisation puts an additional constraint on double helical structure, and the DNA becomes supercoiled (Fig.). One supercoil is introduced every time the duplex thread is twisted about its axis. This supercoiling places a DNA molecule under torsion, which can be released by a break in one of the two strands. A DNA molecule without supercoiling is said to be relaxed.

The supercoils may be negative (as found in vivo), when they are in a direction opposite to the clockwise turns of right handed DNA. This will actually relieve the torsion and will become underwound or even single stranded in a region. This helps in unwinding of DNA for replication, etc. The positive supercoils lead to overwinding (superhelical), which can be created in vitro, but does not occur in nature. Supercoiling is often controlled by some enzymes and is described by parameters like linking number, twisting number and writhing number (for details, consult Lewin's Genes VI').

Ribonucleic acid (RNA). Although double stranded RNA is not uncommon, mainly RNA is found as single stranded molecules. Chemical analysis shows the following two main differences in the polynucleotide chains of DNA and RNA:

(i) While deoxyribose sugar is found in DNA, in RNA ribose sugar is found. This difference between DNA and RNA is the most important and would distinguish the two under all conditions, (ii) While in DNA, adenine, guanine, thymine and cytosine are the four common bases, in RNA the four bases are adenine, guanine, uracil and cytosine. Since there is a large number of other unusual bases found in RNA as well as in DNA and also since thymine may rarely be found in RNA also, this distinction is not as important as that of sugar molecule. There is yet a third distinction described, *i.e.*, double stranded nature of DNA and single stranded nature of RNA. This distinction is no longer tenable in so far as single stranded DNA (*e.g.* phage $\phi \times 174$, parvovirus) and double stranded RNA (see Table) are now known in a number of cases.

While DNA is perhaps always genetic in nature, RNA is only rarely genetic in nature. This would mean that although the primary function of storing and carrying the genetic information is rarely also associated with RNA in some organisms, but mainly RNA, found in all organisms, would perform different important functions during protein synthesis. Therefore, two types of RNA are really known, namely genetic RNA and non-genetic RNA.

Genetic RNA: In most plant viruses, genetic material consists of RNA, although now some plant viruses are known which have DNA. In many bacteriophages also, genetic material is RNA rather than DNA. Viroids and virusoids are other two classes of small RNAs (~350 bases) found in plants. Viroids are subviral pathogens and function independently without encapsidation by a protein coat (*e.g.* potato spindle tuber viroid or PSTV). Virusoids (also called satellite RNAs) are encapsidated by plant viruses packaged together with a viral genome. Virusoids can not replicate independently, and do so with the help of an associated virus. Such genetic RNA contains information which is normally found in DNA in higher organisms. In other words, RNA has replaced DNA in such cases. The RNA found in these viruses could be single stranded or double stranded (Table). When RNA is double stranded, it generally follows the same rules of base pairing as in case of DNA. Different viruses having single stranded or double stranded RNA are listed in Table.

Different RNA Viruses and the Nature of RNA Associated with them

Virus	*Type of RNA*
Plant Viruses	
MV	Single stranded
Wound	Double stranded
Animal Viruses	
Influenza virus	Single stranded
Rous sarcoma	Single stranded
Poliomyelitis	Single stranded
Reovirus	Double stranded
Bacteriophages	
MS2, F2, rl7	Single stranded

Non-genetic RNA. In organisms, where genetic information is contained in, and transmitted through DNA, RNA though present in good quantity, but does not serve as a genetic material. This non-genetic RNA is synthesized on DNA template and is of the following three different types.

(i) Messenger RNA (mRNA) carries genetic information contained in DNA and makes a small fraction (5%-10%) of total RNA present in the cell. This species of RNA is rather short-lived and therefore has a rather rapid turnover. The molecular weight of this RNA varies, usually from 500,000 to 2,000,000.

(ii) Transfer RNA (tRNA), also known as soluble RNA (sRNA), makes another small fraction (10%-15%) of RNA. These are the smallest molecules of RNA and work as adapter molecules for carrying amino acid molecules to the site of protein synthesis. Being smallest in size, these molecules have been most thoroughly investigated.

(iii) Ribosomal RNA (rRNA) is the most stable kind of RNA and is associated with the ribosomes, of which this RNA species makes 40-60 per cent by weight. This species of RNA also makes about 80 per cent of the total RNA in the cell.

Besides the above three major classes of RNA, there is a variety of other non-genetic RNA species found in cells for specific functions. These include the following: (i) Anti-sense RNA also called mic RNA (messenger RNA inhibiting complementary RNA) is synthesized sometimes on the strand complementary to the one used for *m*RNA synthesis. This is used for regulation of DNA synthesis and gene expression both in vivo and in vitro. (ii) HnRNA is synthesized from split genes in eukaryotes, and particular class (group 1) of intron sequences are self-spliced due to ribozyme activity of RNA. (iii) SnRNA (small nuclear RNA), SnoRNA (small nucleolar RNA) and ScRNA (small cytoplasmic RNA) are found in the nucleus, nucleolus and cytoplasm respectively. SnRNAs (Ul, U2, U4, U5, U6) are used for the formation of spliceosome leading to splicing of another category (group 2) of intron sequences, (iv) Guide RNA (gRNA), synthesized from minicircle mitochondrial DNA (*m*DNA), is used for RNA editing leading to modification of RNA transcribed from DNA template.

The Proteins

Different genes in an organism are generally expressed through proteins which are synthesized through the information stored in genes. It is through these proteins that phenotype is eventually determined. There are, of course, some genes which do not express through synthesis of proteins, but are meant for the synthesis of different components of proteins synthesis apparatus. For instance, there are separate genes for different transfer RNA (tRNA) molecules and also for ribosomal RNA (rRNA). These genes do not contain any information for the sequence of amino acids in a protein. In this chapter, a brief introduction only about the structure of proteins will be presented.

Protein Structure

Structure of proteins can be discussed at four levels of organisations: (i) primary structure, (ii) secondary structure, (iii) tertiary structure, and (iv) quaternary structure.

Primary Structure of Proteins: Proteins are polymers of amino acids and at primary level these can be considered to be polypeptide chains in the same manner, as the nucleic acids are known to be polynucleotides (Table).

A Comparison of the Primary Structure of Nucleic Acids and Proteins

Features	*Nucleic Acid*	*Protein*
1. Polymer	Polynucleotide	Polypeptide
2. Basic units	Four types of nucleotides	Twenty essential amino acids listed
	(a) in DNA-pAdR, pTdR, pCdR, pGR	in Table all these amino acids
	(b) in RNA-pAR, pUR, pCR, pGR protein.	need not to be present in a particular
3. Polarity	A polynucleotide chain has a polarity (5' and 3' end)	A polypeptide would have a free-COOH group at one end and a free-NH_2 group at the other end (C-terminal end and N-terminal ends)
Linkage	The nucleotides are linked with the help of 'phospho diester' bonds (-O-P-O-)	The amino acids are linked with the -help of 'peptide' bonds (-CO-NH-)

The polymer (polypeptide) in a protein consists of amino acids linked with the help of peptide (-CO-NH) bonds. The peptide bond consists of a covalent bond between carboxyl group of one amino acid and amino group of another, shown in Figure. The protein backbone consists of the repeating series of alpha carbons, carboxyl carbons and amino nitrogen.

Secondary Structure of Proteins: A polypeptide chain always has a spatial (in space) organisation. The configuration of backbone of polypeptide chain would mean the secondary structure of protein, of which a particular protein may be a part. These secondary structures fall into three main categories: (i) helices (mainly the alpha helix) which can be left handed or right handed (Fig.), (ii) beta strands (backbone is extended or stretched out) or beta sheets (where two or more beta strands are arranged in rows (Fig.) and (iii) turns connecting the helices and strands (beta turns and omega turns). These three secondary elements are shown in Figure.

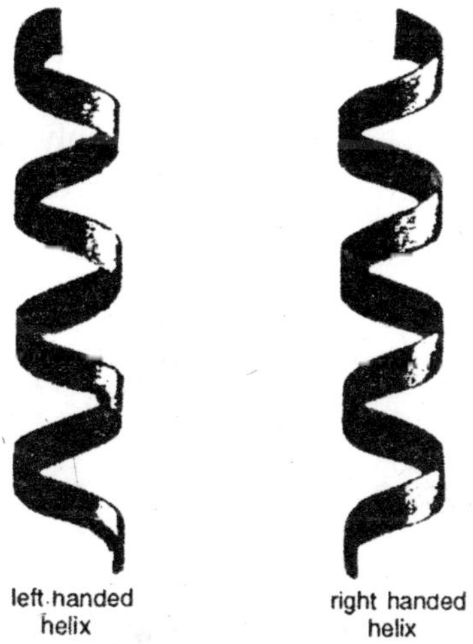

A comparison of a left handed helix and a right handed helix (as a memory device, remember that screws which insert when turned clockwise are right handed and the other is left handed).

The secondary structures are often stabilised by intramolecular hydrogen bonding. These secondary elements can also combine with one another to form motifs, or supersecondary structures, which assemble in the form of a tertiary structure.

$$H_2\ N.\ CH_2\ CO\ \boxed{OH + H}\ NH.\ CH_2\ COOH$$

glycine

$$\longrightarrow H_2\ N.\ CH_2\ CO.NH.CH_2\ COOH$$

↑

depeptide

Formation of a peptide bond between two molecul   n amino acid to form a dipeptide.

Tertiary Structure of Proteins and Second Half of the Genetic Code: Tertiary structure refers to three dimensional structure of a protein. While the secondary structure is obtained by folding and intramolecular bonding in polypeptide, tertiary structure is stabilised by side chains of amino acids.

This three-dimensional structure is important, since it forms sites of specific activity, particularly in case of enzymes. An enzyme would lose its specific activity only through alterations in tertiary structure of protein by whatever factors it is brought about.

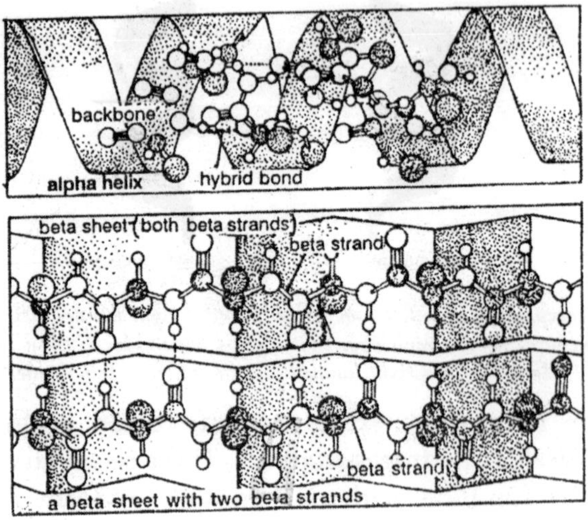

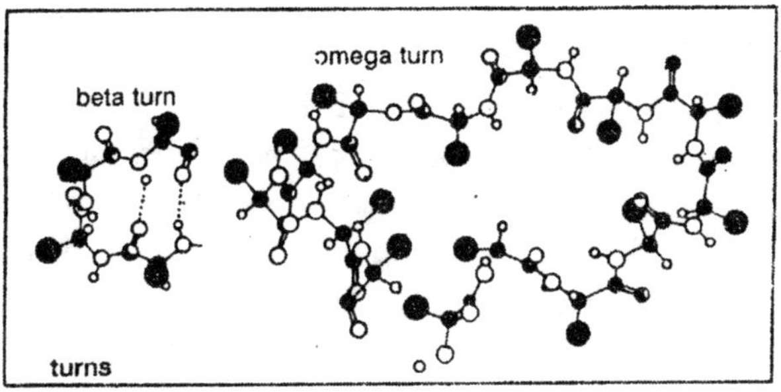

Common secondary structures of proteins (helix, beta sheet and turns).

It has been shown repeatedly that the primary structure of a protein (or in other words the amino acid sequence) is sufficient to specify the tertiary structure of a molecule. However, it is not yet possible to predict the tertiary structure of a protein from its amino acid sequence, because the rules which govern the transformation of a particular amino acid sequence into a specific tertiary structure are not fully understood so far.

Hundreds of laboratories around the world are busy working on this problem, which is often described as protein folding problem or also as second half of the genetic code.

Quaternary Structure of Proteins: Primary, secondary and tertiary structures have been discussed with respect to single polypeptide units. However, in a particular protein, more than one polypeptides may be associated to give rise to a complex macromolecule, which is biologically a functional unit. This structure obtained through combination of more than one polypeptides would be quaternary structure.

Polypeptide units of this quaternary structure would have their own primary, secondary and tertiary structures. It is important to know that, while the mechanism of synthesis of polypeptides (primary structure) is now known in considerable detail, little is known about how particular secondary, tertiary and quaternary structures can be achieved by polypeptides.

Structure of Proteins and Weak Bonds

The most stable arrangement of a polypeptide backbone is a helix, 5.4 Å long. In proteins there is a regular pattern of hydrogen bonds between carbonyl and imino groups on the same chain. There are 3.6 amino acids per turn, providing precise geometry of the polypeptide chain (four amino acids per turn will not allow hydrogen bonds to be so neatly formed). Other favourable arrangements of polypeptide backbone are sheets, where adjacent amino acids are related by 180° rotation (Fig.), so that their side groups are projected in opposite directions. Hydrogen bonds are formed in these sheets between carbonyl and imino groups of either the different chains or of the very distant parts of the same chain bringing two parts of the same chain together as sheets due to two fold symmetry. Two different forms of sheets are known, in one the two adjacent chain run in the same direction (parallel β sheet) and in the second the two chains run in opposite directions (antiparallel β sheets).

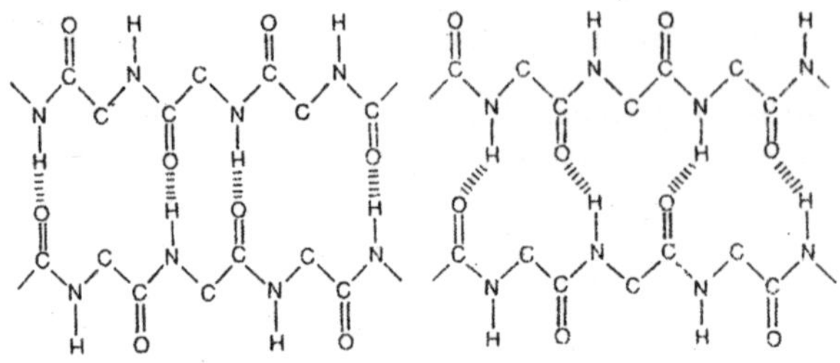

Two B sheets (an antiparallel and a paralleled B Sheet)

It should also be realised that polypeptide chains are not mere polymers of identical monomers forming helices or sheets, but invariably have irregular side groups attached to the backbone. This necessitates a compromise between regular helix or sheet backbone and the tendency of the side groups to twist the backbone into much less regular configurations. This maximises the strength of secondary bonds formed by side groups. In solutions, proteins containing large number of nonpolar side groups tend to be more stable than those containing polar groups. This is because disruption, of molecules with nonpolar group causes much greater loss in free energy than the disruption of molecules with polar groups (disrupted polar groups can make hydrogen bonds with water).

Almost 50 per cent of amino acid residues in proteins do have nonpolar side groups that interact with each other rather than with polar side groups or with water molecules. Within a cell, the proteins assume configurations which allow isolation of nonpolar side group to areas where water can not penetrate (hydrophobic areas).

Ramachandran Plots and Protein Folding

Although, one can not yet predict the three dimensional structure of a protein from its amino-acid sequence, protein structure can be reduced to a few elements or motifs, which are arranged in different ways in different proteins. Further, each of the motif can be further understood in terms of the conformational possibilities of the amino acids. Several chemical characteristics determine the motifs. For instance, studies have shown that the six atoms of the peptide group should all be in the same plane, a feature described as planarity of the peptide bond (Fig.).

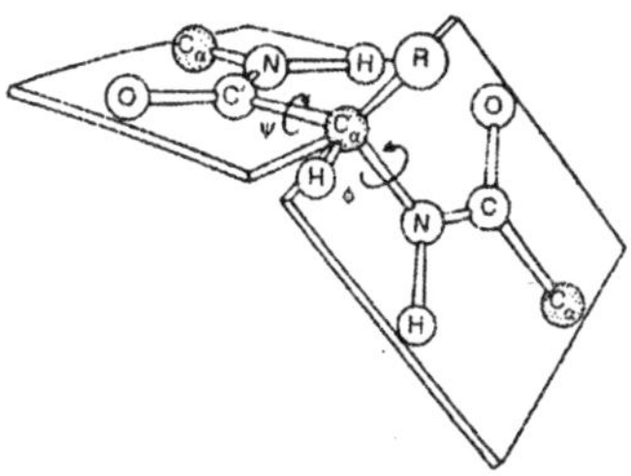

Chemical structure of the peptide bond; partial double bond nature of the peptide bond gives a planar peptide unit, so that the conformation of the protein backbone can be specified in terms of torsion (rotation) angles ϕ and ψ (redrawn from Balasubramanian et. al. Concepts in Biotechnology', 1996)

However, some degree of rotation is allowed about the bonds, which join the peptide groups to the α -carbon atom. These rotations are designated as torsion angles ϕ and ψ . The values of ϕ and ψ are influenced to different degrees due to steric hindrance from the side chains. The permissible range of ϕ and ψ can be plotted against each other to give what are popularly described as Ramachandran plots (Fig.). Some of the values of ϕ and ψ can give regular patterns of atoms, if they are repeated over a number of residues in the protein chain. These patterns are actually the secondary structures. The Ramachandran plots are so called after the name of Professor G.N. Ramachandran, who worked at the Department of Crystallography and Biophysics, University of Madras and later at Indian Institute of Science, Bangalore. He became internationally known for his seminal work in the area of structural biophysics. One of the important contributions of Professor Ramachandran was his correct proposal of the triple helical structure of the fibrous protein, collagen (Fig.).

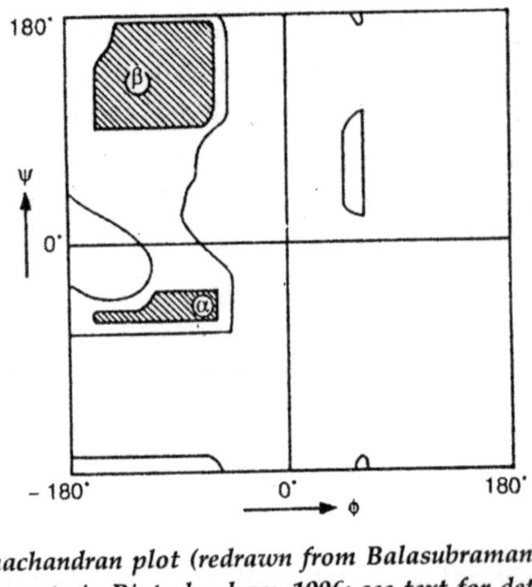

The Ramachandran plot (redrawn from Balasubramanian et. al., Concepts in Biotechnology, 1996; see text for details)

Professor G.N. Ramachandran and his group studied the conformational possibilities inherent in a polypeptide chain. These possibilities were based on the following valid assumptions: (i) the peptide bond is rigid and will not allow rotation; (ii) the molecule may be rotated about the other single bonds in the backbone, *i.e.*, the N-C_α bond and C_α - C′ bonds; (iii) all atoms are represented as hard spheres, there being no chance of inter-penetration (even though we know that atoms are not spheres, but for this purpose they were treated as hard spheres); (iv) there are no other attractive or repulsive forces.

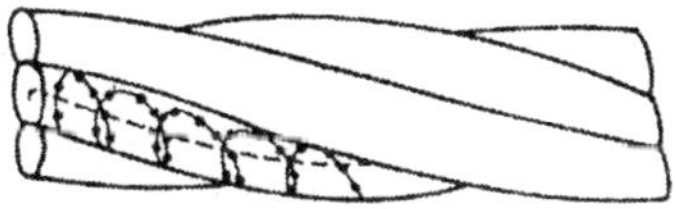

A triple helix representing collagen (redrawn from Balasubramanian et. al. Concepts in Biotechnology, 1996)

Based on the above assumptions, conformational possibilities of a dipeptide can be represented in the form of a 'Ramachandran map' shown in the Figure. The hatched areas represent the combinations of ϕ and ψ torsion angles allowed for any dipeptide (other than glycine, which has a much larger region allowed, since it is the smallest of the amino acids). These regions expanded a bit, when inter-penetration of the atomic spheres were accepted later. These Ramachandran plots did not change very much over the last more than three decades, during which thousands of proteins were found to have 98 per cent of their residues well within the limits suggested in Ramachandran plots. The values of ϕ and ψ which if repeated in consecutive residues (and thus leading to regular structures), are also marked in the map (a helix and (3 sheets). Some of these secondary structures are described in terms of ϕ and ψ.

α-helix: When (ϕ, ψ) values (-57°,-47°) are repeated, the polypeptide backbone chain of the protein is folded in a right-handed manner around an axis giving it the appearance of a helix with side chains extending out. This a helix is stabilised by hydrogen bonds, which are formed between C - O group of each amino acid and - N - H group of amino acid situated four residues ahead in the linear sequence. Each residue is related to the next one by 1.5Å along the axis and a rotation of 100° about it, thus giving 3.6 amino acid residues per turn and a pitch of 5.4 A (3.6 x 1.5 = 5.4) and a radius of 2.3Å. (example : keratin protein in hairs or wool).

The β Strand and β Pleated Sheet: When the backbone of a polypeptide chain is extended or stretched out, it forms, what is described as β strand. The extended polypeptide chains can also associate by hydrogen bonds to form sheet like structures. These structures are planar and the polypeptide chains involved may be parallel or antiparallel.

These are called β sheets. The distance between adjacent residues, along the direction of the sheet is 3.5Å. Hydrogen bond between N - H and C - O of different polypeptide chains stabilise the structure. The silk fibre exist in β-shrand or β-sheet, which gives the silk its tensile strength.

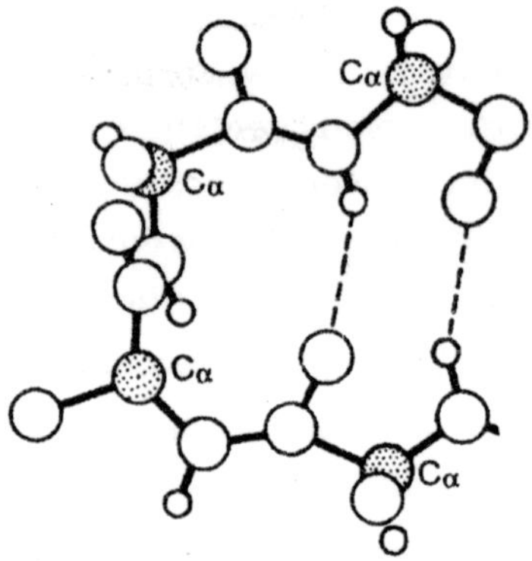

A β-turn conformation (redrawn from Balasubramanian et. al., Concepts in Biotechnology, 1996)

β turns (or reverse turns) and ω (omega) turns). The polypeptide chain sometimes reverses its direction, and it does so with the help of a structural motif called P turn or reverse turn or omega turn (Fig.). Such turns are abundantly formed in proteins, particularly in globular proteins. Turns sometimes also connect helices and strands as in the Rossmann fold (Fig.) giving rise to a supersecondary structure.

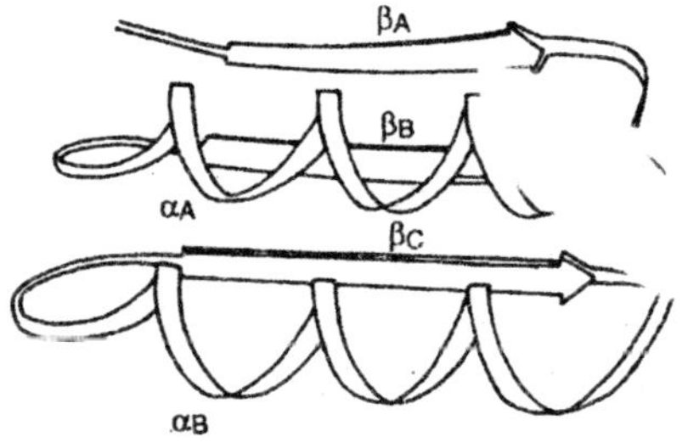

The Rossmann fold, a common supersecondary structural unit. It alternates between α β strand and an α helix along the chain; the β strands are arranged in a sheet, and α helices are held together (redrawn from Balasaburamnian et. al., Concepts in Biotechnology, 1996)

Protein Conformation Based Inheritance: The Prions

As discussed earlier in this chapter among cellular macromolecules, nucleic acids are known, to be the sole hereditary determinants. However, during 1980's and 1950's, cases have been reported, where proteins were shown to determine inheritance through conformational changes. This is popularly described now as "protein conformation based inheritance," although some workers believe that the evidence in favour of this type of inheritance is not uncquivocal. This protein conformation based inheritance is exhibited by infectious particles called "prions". The term 'prion' was introduced in 1982 by Stanley B Prusiner of the University of California (San Francisco), who has been awarded the 1997 Nobel Prize in Medicine. The term was used to characterise the proteinaceous infectious particles causing a variety of mammalian neurodegenerative diseases which are generally fatal and are referred to as transmissible spongiform encephalopathies (TSEs). These include diseases like Scrapie, CJD (Creutzfeldt-Jakob Disease), GSS (Gertsmann-Straussler-Scheinker Disease) and Kuru.

Prions also cause the 'mad cow disease' or 'bovine spongiform encephalopathy' (BSE), which created a panic in Britain in 1996, since the disease was suspected to be caused due to eating BSE-tainted beef.

Despite being infectious, prions differ from viruses, viroids, retroviruses and virusoids or satellite viruses in having no nucleic acid components whatsoever (viruses have their own DNA/RNA and proteins; viroids are RNA molecules not encapsidated; virusoids are nucleic acid molecules encapsulated by protein coat derived from other viruses, and the retroviruses carry cellular oncogenes).

The absence of nucleic acids and presence of only proteins in these pathogens was initially proved, when it was observed that UV and ionizing radiations (which damage nucleic acids) did not cause any loss of infectivity, while treatments involving modification or hydrolysis of proteins caused loss of infectivity.

The prion protein is designated as PrP. Since it occurs both in the normal and the infected hamsters, apparently it can not cause the disease.

Since the protease resistant core of PrP has a molecular weight of 27-30kDa, it is also known as PrP 27-30. This PrP is only a part of a larger protein PrP with a molecular weight of 33-35 kDa (superscript Sc stands for protein causing scrapie), which causes infection.

A subset of PrP is also designated as PrP, which is protease sensitive and works as a substrate for PrP, the essential component of the infectious prion particle. Physically, PrP^{Sc} differs from PrP by its insolubility in detergents, its propensity to aggregate and its relative resistance to proteolysis. While PrP^{c} is rich in α helices, PrP^{Sc} is rich in β sheets (Fig.). Further, unlike PrP^{c} PrP^{Sc} tends to form insoluble aggregates and fibrils in brain cells (Fig.).

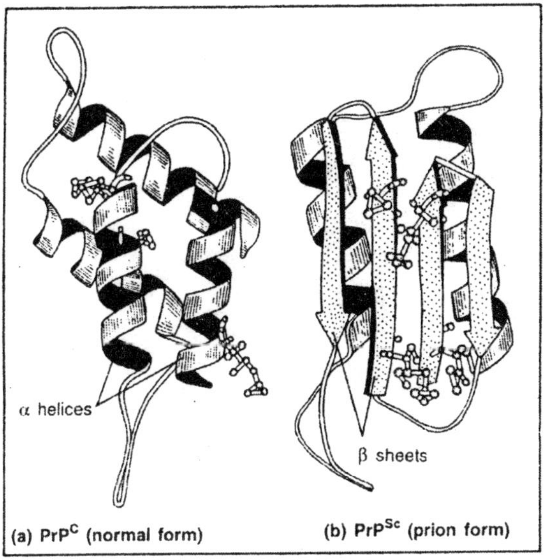

Two conformations of person, PrP^c (rich in α helices) and PrP^{Sc} (rich in β Sheets)

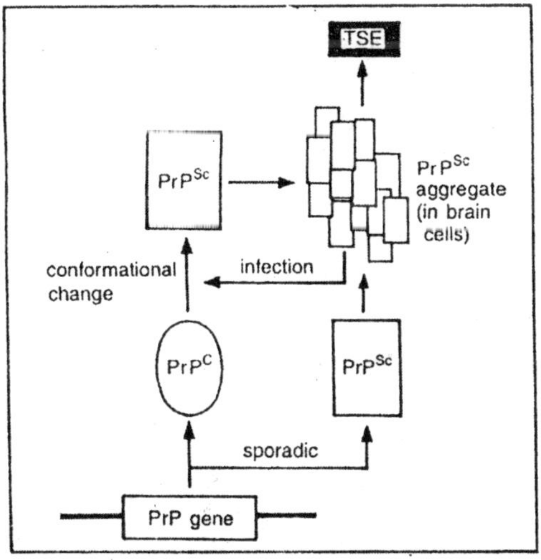

A hypothesis suggesting conformational change in prion protein PrP^c giving rise to P$_r$P^{Sc}, which forms aggregates and fibrils in brain cells causing 'transmissible spongiform encephalopathies' (TSE).

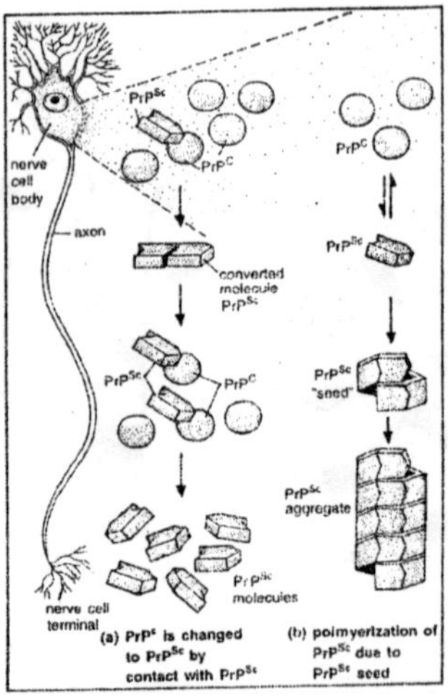

Two models for post-translational conversion of PrPc into PrP^{Sc}.

The prion diseases have also been shown to be hereditary. The PrP gene in Syrian Hamster has two exons, while that of mouse has three exons. However, the open reading frame (ORF) of all the known PrP genes is present in a single exon in each case, so that PrP^{Sc} can not result due to alternative RNA splicing, but should only result due to post translational modification. Several prion diseases are actually caused due to mutations in the PrP genes (P*rn*-P). Genetic nature of prion diseases was also demonstrated by using transgenic mice carrying Prn-P from Syrian Hamster (SHaPrP) and also by ablation of the Prn-P in mice (Prn-P$^{0/0}$). In both these cases it was shown that the de novo synthesis of prion is species specific or transgene specific.

Since there is no evidence available for the presence of scrapie-specific nucleic acid, and since proteins are incapable of undergoing self replication, alternative mechanisms for prion propagation have been proposed. It has been shown that post-translational conversion of PrP^{c} encoded in PrP gene is obligatory for development of prion disease. This conversion can be achieved in one of the following ways (Fig.) (i) PrP^{Sc}

combines with PrP^c to give PrP^c-PrP^{Sc} complex, which changes to PrP^{Sc}-PrP^{Sc}. The homodimer PrP^{Sc}-PrP^{Sc} gives rise to two heterodimers PrP^c-PrP^{Sc}, which again change to two molecules of homodimers (PrP^{Sc}-PrP^{Sc}) thus forming four molecules of PrP^{Sc} and so on; (ii) PrP^c changes to PrP^{Sc} through conformational change from α -helices to β -sheets (PrP^c has a higher β -sheet and lower α -helix content, relative to PrP^c, which has four α -helical domains).

Study of Polysaccharides

We discussed the structure of simple sugars represented by a class of micromolecules. These sugars included monosaccharides and oligosaccharides. Polysaccharides represent a class of macromolecules that contain, each atleast 10 or more monosaccharide units.

They are given names by replacing the ending -ose in the name of their monomers, by -an. For instance, polysaccharides derived from glucose (*e.g.* cellulose) are glucans. Similarly, polysaccharides derived from fructose are called fructans. A general name for polysaccharides is glycan, because monosaccharides are given the general name glucose. The popular names starch, cellulose, pectin, amylopectin, inulin, chitin and heparin are still used, although they do not conform to the above nomenclature, where all poly-saccharides should have names ending with '-an'.

Polysaccharides have been classified into two groups: (i) homopolysaccharides (also called homoglycans) containing only one type of monosaccharide or glycose units and (ii) heteropolysaccharides (also called heteroglyeans) containing atleast two different monosaccharides (or glycose) units (Table). Most heteropoly-saccharides do not contain more than two types of glycose units. These polysaccharides are formed due to condensation of many molecules of monosaccharides with simultaneous release of water molecules. Because each monosaccharide has several free hydroxyl groups that can be used for condensation with another monosaccharide, the number of possible structures of a polysaccharide involving the same monosaccharide units, can be large. Three hexoses ($C_6H_{12}O_6$) can join in a variety of ways to give thousands of different trisaccharides and so on.

In view of this, it is extremely difficult to determine the structure of a polysaccharide, because this will involve the determination of the sites of linkage between every two adjacent monosaccharide units. Consequently, it has been shown to be much more difficult to determine the structure of a polysaccharide than to determine the nucleotide sequence in a nucleic acid molecule or to determine the amino acid sequence in a protein.

Homopolysaccharides (Homoglycans)

As mentioned above, homoglycans will consist of same monosaccharide units (*e.g.* glucose, fructose, galactose, mannose, xylose, etc.). The best examples of homo-polysaccharides are glycogen in animals and starch and cellulose in plants. All of them are composed of only glucose residues. While glycogen and starch are used for storing energy, cellulose makes the extracellular matrix (ECM) or cell wall in plants. Different homopolysaccharides, their repeat units and the linkage type in each case are summarised in Table.

Starch and Glycogen: Starch is the reserved food in plant cells and is a polymer of D-glucopyranose units linked by α-1, 4 linkages (occasionally α-1, 6 linkages are found in amylopectin giving it a branched structure). It consists of amylose and amylopectin in the ratio of 1 : 4. While amylose has a linear structure (200-500 glucose units; mol. wt. ~ 1500,000), amylopectin has a branched structure (1000 glucose residues; mol. wt. ~ 200,000 to 1000,000 (Figs.). If starch is mixed in hot water, only amylose is dissolved and not the amylopectin. Glycogen is the major reserve carbohydrate in animals and is, therefore, sometimes called animal starch. It is mainly found in liver and muscles. The glycogen in the liver supplies glucose to all tissues through the blood, while that in the muscle is used during muscle contraction. Glycogen consists of only glucose

Different Classes of Polysaccharides

Class of Polysaccharide	*Linkage*
1. Homopolysaccharides (homoglycans)	
(a) Glucans (glucose)	
Starch	α -1,4
Glycogen	α -1,4; α -1,6
Cellulose	β - 1,4
Chitin	β - 1, 4
(b) Galactans (galactose)	
Agar	
Pectin	
Galactan	
(c) Mannans (mannan)	α — 1,6
(d) Xylans (xylose)	5-1,4
(hemicellulose xylan)	
(e) Fructans, *e.g.*, inulin (fructose)	β - 1, 2
2. Heteropolysaccharides	
(heteroglycans)	—
(a) Neutral sugars	
(several monomers)	

Contd...

Class of Polysaccharide	*Linkage*
(b) Mucopolysaccharides	
Hyaluronic acid (disaccharide)	β —1,4
Chondroitin sulphates (disaccharide)	β-1,4
Heparin (disaccharide)	—
3. Other heteropolysaccharides (sugars linked to other molecules)	
(a) Glycoproteins (sugars linked to peptides)	—
(b) Lipoproteins (sugars linked to lipids)	—

* repeat units are given in parentheses

units (5000-15,000 in a molecule) linked by α -1, 4 and α -1, 6 linkages giving it a branched structure with a molecular weight ranging from 300,000 to 100×10^6.

Cellulose: It is the most important constituent of the extracellular matrix (cell wall) in plants. It is insoluble in most solvents and thus differ from starch and glycogen. It is a linear polymer with β-1, 4 glycosidic bonds, where a number of linear chains are held together to form microfibrillar. It can be hydrolysed by cellulase found in some snails, termites, and the bacteria found in the rumen of cattle and other ruminants.

Heteropolysaccharides (Heteroglycans)

Heteropolysaccharides consist of more than one monosaccharides. Sometimes, the repeating unit is a disaccharide. Heteropolysaccharides can be of the following two types.

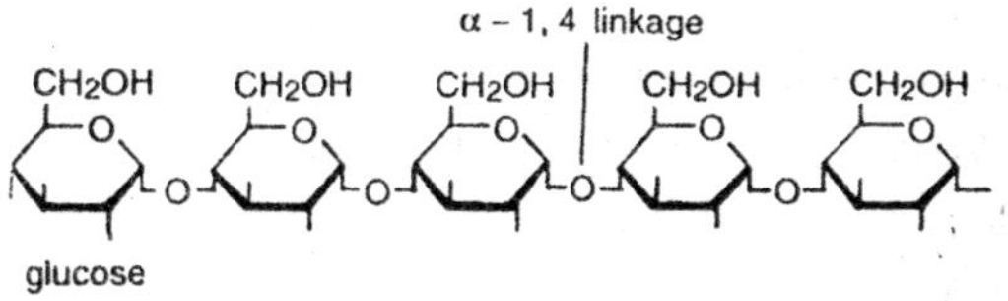

(a) structure of amylose showing α– 1,4 linkage

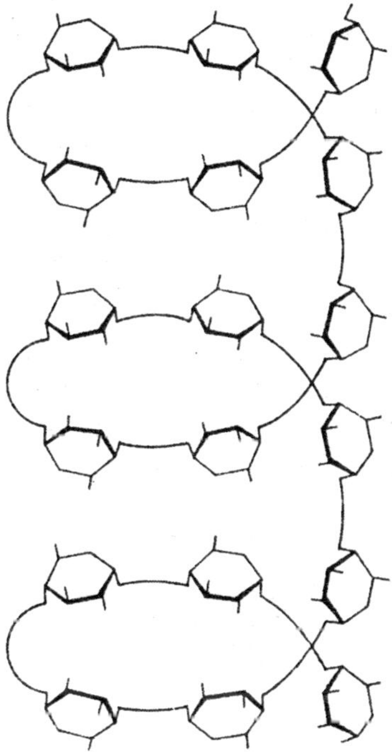

(b) helical coil of amylose on suspension in water

Linear structure of amylose.

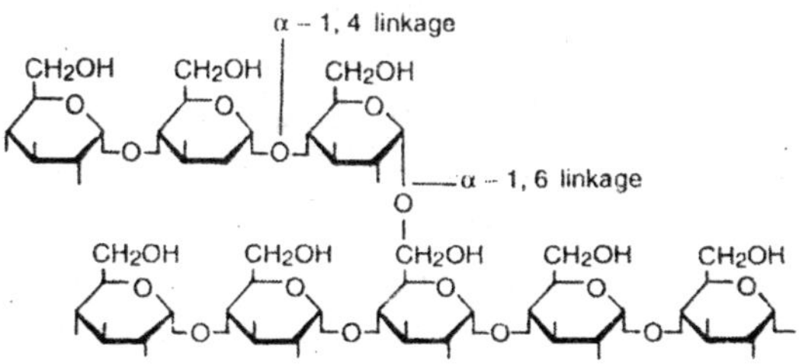

Branched structure of amylopectin.

Neutral Sugars: They include hemicelluloses, gums, mucilages and pectic substances. They contain a number of different sugars (*e.g.* xylose, arbinose, galactose, rhamnose, mannose, glucuronic acid, etc.) and also some non-sugar compounds.

Mucopolysaccharides: They consist of amino sugars, uronic acids and some of their derivatives. Generally they are structural polysaccharides and are found in the connective tissues of animals (*e.g.* blood). Following are the three main examples of mucopolysaccharides: (i) Hyaluronic acid is found in skin, vitreous humour of the eye, the umbilical cord, etc. It is a linear polymer of disaccharide repeat units linked with the help of β-1, 4 glycosidic bonds. In a disaccharide repeat unit there are two monosaccharides-D-glucuronic acid and N-acetyl-D-glucosamine, linked using β-1,3 bond, (ii) Chondroitin sulphates are found in cornea, cartilage, tendons, skin, heart, saliva, etc. The repeating unit is a disaccharide consisting of glucuronic acid and sulphate ester of N-acetyl galactosamine, linked through a β-1, 3 bond. The disaccharides are linked with each other by β-1, 4 bonds, (iii) Heparin is secreted by most cells in the intestinal mucosa, liver, lung, spleen and kidney. It is an anticoagulant and is used in blood banks for preventing clotting of blood.

Glycoproteins and Glycolipids

Polysaccharides are also found associated with proteins and lipids, so that they are then described as glycoproteins and glycolipids. These sugar rich molecules make a sugar rich zone on the surface of plasma membrane, which is described as glycocalyx. A glycoprotein consists of a polysaccharide linked to a polypeptide by a covalent bond. Most of the soluble and membrane bound proteins that are made in the ER are glycoproteins. These are sometimes transported from ER to Golgi apparatus, lysosomes, plasma membrane and extracellular space. The sugar component of these glycoproteins is generally the same in all such glycoproteins. It consists of 14 sugar residues and the association between sugar and protein is facilitated by oligosaccharyl transferase. This polysaccharide consisting of 14 residues is linked to the NH_2 group of an asparagine (N) amino acid in the protein, hence described as N-linked or asparagine-linked (Fig.).

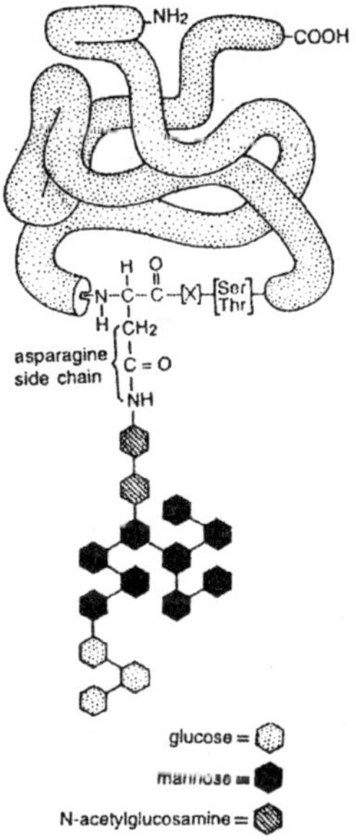

An N-linked or asparagine linked oligosaccharide, (O-linked glycosylation also takes place in some proteins; O stands for serine or threonine), that is added to most proteins in the rough ER membrane (redrawn from Alberts et. al. Molecular Biology of the cell, 1994)

Glycolipids are also found in the non-cytoplasmic half of the lipid bilayer in all animal membranes, thus making their distribution asymmetric. These glycolipids work as receptors and also help a cell to bind to its own extracellular matrix (ECM) and to the other cells. The most complex of these glycolipids are gangliosides, which contain oligosaccharides with one or more sialic acid residues. These gangliosides are most abundant in the nerve cells.

4

Role of Walls

Cell Walls

The presence of cell wall in plants and its absence in animal cells is generally described as a major distinction between plant and animal cells. However, it is now known that although, the cell wall, as a mechanically rigid and rather porous structure, is absent in animal cells, a corresponding structure (not rigid like the cell wall) is present outside the plasma membrane of animal cells also. Consequently, a common term has been used (both in animal and plant cells) for the structures present outside the plasma membrane. This structure making the outermost boundary of the cell, both in animals and plants is described as extracellular matrix (ECM). Therefore the cell, wall in higher plants actually represents a unique type of extracellular matrix, having both structural and growth regulating functions.

The cell wall in bacteria consists of carbohydrates and lipids and the cell wall in plants consists of cellulose, hemicellulose and compounds of pectic acid. In contrast, the ECM in animals consists of proteins and polysaccharides secreted locally and assembled into an organised mesh work in close association with the surface of the cell. The cell walls of plants are generally thick, strong and rigid structures, which envelope the cells including the plasma membranes. It is due to these rigid structures that Robert Hooke in 1663, could distinguish structures in a cork, which he called cells.

The extracellular matrix (including the cell wall) is involved in a variety of functions including the following: (i) transport of a variety of materials on either side ; (ii) recognition of a variety of stimuli with the help of receptor proteins and (iii) cell adhesions (including cell-cell adhesions and attachment to the substratum). The structure of extracellular matrix and its above functions have been the subject of active research in recent years, because any defect associated with them leads to serious hereditary diseases. In this chapter we will discuss the structure and function of these outermost envelopes of plant and animal cells.

Extracellular Womb

In plants (including bacteria) a cell is always surrounded by a cell wall lined throughout with plasmalemma. While the bacterial cell wall consists of protein-lipid-polysaccharide complexes, the cell wall of plants mainly consists of cellulose, hemicellulose and compounds of pectic acid. The presence or absence of cell wall is one of the most important distinctions between plants and animals, because the presence or absence of chlorophyll is not as important. Many plants may become heterotrophic due to loss of chlorophyll, but they still have a definite cell wall, which is absent in case of animal cells.

Cell Wall in Bacteria: The outermost boundary or the envelope of a bacterial cell is a complex structure in comparison to their relatively simpler cytosol. The innermost layer of this envelope is always a phospholipid bilayer in which a variety of proteins remains inserted. This is the plasma membrane. Outside this plasma membrane is present the lipid cell wall or the extracellular matrix (ECM). Depending upon the constitution (determined on the basis of their reaction to a staining protocol) of the cell wall, bacteria have been classified into following two types (Figs.); (i) Gram-positive bacteria (*e.g.* Bacillus), characterised by the presence of a rigid shell (periplasmic shell) consisting of carbohydrates and amino acids, which is called peptidoglycan (in plants, this cell wall consists of cellulose, hemicellulose and compounds of pectic acid). (ii) Gram-negative bacteria (*e.g.*, Escherichia coli), characterised by the presence of a second membrane described as 'outer membrane' or as 'outer lipopolysaccharide layer', located outside the thin peptidoglycan layer (inner membrane).

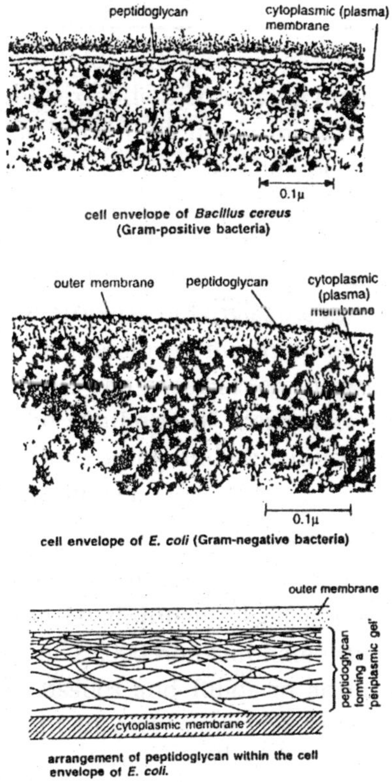

The structure of cell wall in Gram-negative bacteria.

Unlike the rigid and porous cell wall of higher plants, the outer membrane of Gram negative bacteria and the inner membrane (peptidoglycan) of both the types of bacteria contain transport proteins that mediate the passage of selected solutes. In recent years the structure of these bacterial transport proteins has been studied in detail. The structure and function of these bacterial transport proteins.

Cell Wall in Higher Plants

Significance of Cell Wall: During the last two decades (1980-2000), there has been a revolution in our thinking about cell wall. They are no longer considered static and rigid structures as earlier believed, but have, instead, been found to be very dynamic, very porous, very malleable and capable of broadcasting signals to the cells, they come in contact. For instance, in late 1980s, it was shown in the brown alga, Fucus, that if cell wall in young embryo is enzymatically destroyed, the embryo forgets where the rhizoids are supposed to grow and a fresh exposure to light caused the rhizoids to grow in new directions.

The cell wall thus had signals needed to direct root growth. Later, in 1994, it was shown that the destiny of the two cells of a two celled embryo depended on their cell walls. As soon as the cell walls were removed, the cell goes back to zygotic state and could become anything. In the year 1998, it was also shown in Arabidopsis roots that only those epidermal cells which touch the junction between two underlying cortical cells (inside the epidermal layer) are capable of forming root hairs, suggesting the presence of signaling molecules at the junctions of cortical cells. S-locus glycoproteins on the stigma/style are one such class of signaling molecules. Another class of molecules are expansions, that were discovered in 1992, and are known to induce cell growth (for more details, see later).

Cell wall has recently attracted the attention of molecular

biologists for the following two other important reasons also: (i) The cell wall in forages make a major part of forage dry matter, but only 50 per cent of this dry matter is readily digested. Much of, lignin interferes with the digestibility of polysaccharides, thus rendering much of the cellulose and hemicellulose inaccessible to rumen microorganisms; (ii) High proportion of lignin in cell wall, causes problems in paper pulp processing, thus increasing the cost, making the process more complex, and causing environmental hazards (pollution). Therefore, considerable current research effort is also targeted towards reducing the amount of lignin or towards modifying lignin structure, either to improve the digestibility of forage legumes/grasses or to facilitate pulping of trees for paper industry.

Structure of Cell Wall: Structure of cell wall of higher plants may be described under the following sections: (1) middle lamella, (2) primary wall, (3) secondary wall, and (4) tertiary wall.

Middle Lamella: Middle lamella is the outermost layer of plant cell wall and connects the two adjacent cells (Fig.). It is primarily composed of pectic substances. It is also called intercellular substance and differs from other components of cell wall in stainability. It can be dissolved by strong acids.

Primary Wall: Primary wall consists of those layers or wall lamellae which are present on both sides of middle lamella. The layers present on two sides of middle lamella will obviously belong to two different adjacent cells. It is rather difficult to distinguish it from secondary wall except by its position and it would gradually merge into secondary wall. Main distinction between primary wall and secondary wall is due to ontogeny. Since primary wall is laid down first in the ontogeny, it can be clearly seen/ in the newly formed cells. However, primary wall is rather thin and only semi-rigid in comparison to secondary wall.

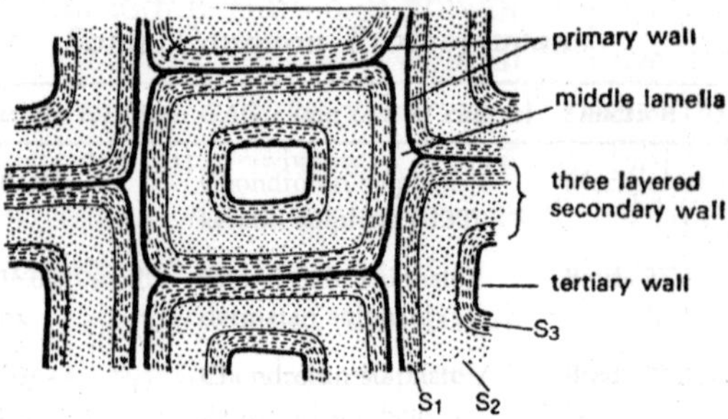

A few cells showing gross structure of cell wall (redrawn from Frey-Wyssling and Muhelthaler: Ultrastructural Plant Cytology, 1965).

The structure of primary cell wall has recently been described in the form of three intermolecular networks: (i) The first network is made "up of the cellulose microfibrils; adjacent microfibrils are connected with the help of xyloglucan chains hydrogen bonded to the surface of these microfibrils, thus forming a continuous lattice. This is embedded in the second network, (ii) The second network consists of pectic polysaccharides, which are rich in uronic acid residues and form cross-links based on calcium bridges and other ionic interactions, (iii) The third interlocking network consists of structural proteins and interweave through the other two domains forming the 'wart and weft' structure. The cellulose microfibrils are embedded in the matrix composed of hemicellulose and pectic material.

Secondary Wall: Secondary wall, which is deposited after the primary wall is laid down, is much thicker and consists of several layers, so that bulk of cell wall at maturity consists of secondary wall only. It is through this secondary wall that the cell attains its shape and in many kinds of cells, this part gives the mechanical strength. In tracheids of conifers, for instance, secondary wall appears to be divided into three layers termed as S_1,S_2 and S_3 (Fig.). In cases like this, primary wall is so thin that it cannot be easily distinguished from the middle lamella. Of the three layers of secondary wall, S_2 is relatively very thick.

Tertiary Wall: Tertiary wall is rarely present and is found on inner side of secondary wall. This is really a dried up residue of degenerated plasma lining. Whether the so-called tertiary wall should be considered a part of the cell wall can be debated, but it has some of the properties shared by primary wall.

Infrastructure and Chemical Composition of Cell Wall: Cell wall when studied with the help of an electron microscope after maceration, is found to consist of two main parts, namely (i) the microfibrils which are left, if hemicellulose and pectic materials are removed and (ii) the ground substance or matrix in which the microfibrils remain embedded (Fig.). Chemically, the cell wall consists of the following major constituents; (i) polysaccharides including cellulose and hemicellulose, (ii) polysaccharides including pectin, (iii) proteins, (iv) lignin (aromatic compounds), (v) ions and (vi) water. Of these the first four are more important and will be discussed in some detail.

Cellulose and Hemicelluloses: The main chemical component of the cell wall is cellulose, which is the most abundant polymer found in nature. A cellulose molecule consists of atleast 500 glucose residues, that are covalently linked to form a ribbon like structure, which is stabilised by hydrogen bonds within a chain. Intermolecular hydrogen bonds between adjacent cellulose molecules cause them to adhere strongly to one another in an overlapping manner. This leads to formation of bundles of 60-70 cellulose chains, all having the same polarity.

These bundles are described as 'cellulose microfibrils', each several micrometers (μ m) long and 3.5nm in diameter, and arranged in a layer of lamellae. Each microfibril is spaced 20-40nm from its neighbour, which are connected with each other through long 'hemicellulose molecules' that make hydrogen bonds with the surface of the microfibrils. The hemicellulose molecules are a heterogeneous group of branched polysaccharides, which are not only bound to microfibrils, but also to one another thus making a hemicellulose complex network. There are many classes of hemicelluloses, but each of them has a long linear backbone composed of one type of sugar, from which short side chains of other sugars protrude. The sugars in the backbone and the side-chains vary according to plant species. The hydrogen bonds between cellulose microfibrils and the hemicelluloses involve only the sugars on the backbone of these hemicelluloses.

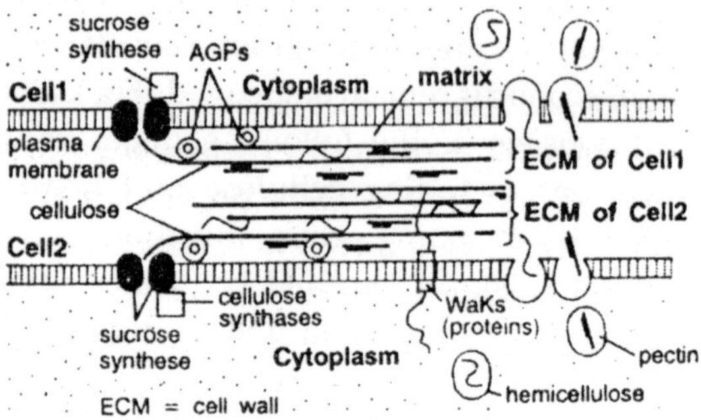

A part of matrix of cell wall, showing fibrillar network

Pectin: In addition to the complex network involving cellulose microfibrils and hemicelluloses as above, in the cell walls of higher plants, there is another 'network of pectins' consisting of cross-linked polysaccharides. Pectins are also a heterogeneous group of branched polysaccharides that generally contain many negatively charged galacturonic acid (GalUA) residues. Because of their negative charge, pectins are hydrated and remain associated with cations, which make cross-links with them. Pectin polysaccharides actually exist in the cell wall in either of the two following forms;

(i) they may form 'smooth regions' of a linear copolymer of α -(l-4)- linked galacturonic acid (GalUA) or

(ii) they may form 'hairy regions', that have attached α -(l-2)-l inked rhamnosyl residues. Pectic polysaccharides are rapidly and extensively degraded from wall matrices (unlike lignin). They form significant portion of cell wall in forage legumes reaching upto 100-300 μg g^{-1} in alfalfa (only 10 μg g~ or less in grasses) and their proportion can be further increased to improve forage disgestibility.

Proteins: In the primary cell walls, there are also proteins, some of them having high levels of hydroxyproline, like collagen. These proteins strengthen the cell wall and are produced locally in abundance, whenever there is an attack by microorganisms. These are also produced during differentiation to modify cells according to local needs.

Lignin, Suberin, Cutin, etc.: In secondary cell walls, additional substances may be incorporated. These include lignin and suberin. Lignins are the second most abundant polymer (after cellulose) found in nature, and are often defined as "phenolic-derived aromatic polymers", that interact with other wall polymers to provide structural integrity, resistance to degradation and water impermeability.

During the last decade (1900-2000), the understanding of the structure and function of lignin has greatly advanced. They are derived, mainly from three primary precursors (coniferyl alcohol, sinapyl alcohol and p-coumaryl alcohol) due to dehydrogenative polymerisation.

Lignins provide structural support for land plants and work as mechanical barrier for imparting pest resistance. But lignin negatively affects processing of pulp in paper industry (cost, complexity and pollution) and also the disgestibility of feed for livestock. Consequently, although lignin serves some vital function for the plants, but adversely affects the utility of plant products for human consumption.

Therefore, if the quantity of lignin in the cell walls is reduced, sizable economic benefits will be derived from this.

In order to meet this objective, considerable effort has already been targeted towards reducing the amount of lignin or towards modification of lignin structure to facilitate pulping of trees and improving digestibility of forage crops.

Transgenic plants have been produced to identify genes for many steps in lignin biosynthesis pathway, and provided important insight into how lignin content can be reduced or its structure modified (more details about this aspect are beyond the scope of this book).

In cell walls of epidermal cells, cutin and cutin waxes may produce impermeable surface coating, checking water loss. In many fungi, cell wall is composed of chitin, a polymer of glucosamine. Substances found in primary and secondary walls are listed in Table, along with their chemical nature and staining reactions.

Comparison of Cell Wall in Dicots and Commelinoid Monocots: Analysis of primary cell wall in monocotyledons and dictyledons suggested that the composition of primary cell wall in 'commelinoid' group of monocotyledon families ('commelinoid' group includes about half of the monocotyledon families including the grasses) differ from that of the primary cell wall of other monocotyledons and dicotyledons (Table). The cell wall in commelinoid group contains ferulic acid and have glucuronoarabinoxylans as one of the major non-cellulosic polysaccharides.

Further, the cell walls in grasses differ from those in other commelinoids in containing another polysaccharide, 1, 3; 1, 4-β glucans. In contrast, the primary cell walls of non-commelinoid monocotyledons have a composition similar to that of primary cell wall of most dicotyledons; they do not contain ferulic acid and have pectic polysaccharides, together with xyloglucans as the major group of non-cellulosic polysaccharides.

Chemical Composition of Plant Cell Walls

Substances	*Chemical unit*	*Staining reaction*
1. Cellulose	Glucose	Chlorzine iodide (stains violet)
2. Hemicellulose	Arabinose, xylose mannose and galactose	None specific
3. Pectin	Glucuronic and	Ruthenium red galacturonic acids
4. Lignin	Coniferyl alcohol	Phloroglucinol hydrochloride (stains rose) ; chlorzine iodide (stains yellow)
5. Cuticular	Fatty acids substances	Sudan III (stains orange)
6. Mineral deposits	Ca and Mg as carbonates or silicates	—

Differences in Composition of Primary Cell Wall in Commelinoid Monocotyledons and Other Flowering Plants.

Class of components	*Commelinoid monocotyledons*	*Non-commelinoid monocotyledons + dicotyledons*
1. Non-cellulosic polysacchari des	Glucuronoarabino-xylans, 1,3; 1, 4-β glucans (only grasses)	Xyloglucans, pectic polysaccharides
2. Ferulic acid	Present	Absent

Functions of Cell Wall, Cell Wall Provides Mechanical Strength: The function of cell wall in plants were earlier believed mainly to provide mechanical strength. More recently, the cell walls have been shown to be more dynamic, even broadcasting signals to other cells. Particularly in higher plants having vascular system, cell walls provide main supporting framework. Since in animals, some sort of exoskeleton or endoskeleton is present, perhaps there is hardly any necessity of definite cell walls. Therefore besides others, main function of the cell wall is the same as that of a skeleton in animals.

Tensile Stress, Stress Relaxation and Cell Expansion: The cell wall in plants controls the size and shape of cells. Structure of cell wall can be stabilised by deposition of lignin. This is required in connection with transition from aquatic to terrestrial plant life, where more mechanical strength is needed. The lignified cell wall consists of microfibrils embedded in matrix consisting of lignin. The cell wall is under considerable tensile stress by the internal hydrostatic pressure of the cell but is quite rigid to resist this pressure, which can reach to the level of about 10 atmospheres. Therefore, the cell wall provides a formidable barrier to the increase in volume of the cell. Despite this, the plant cell does expand by a factor of 10 to 100 times the original volume during maturation. This enlargement of the cell is initiated by stress relaxation of the wall, which leads to water uptake by the cell and surface expansion of the wall. As water enters, the protoplast expands, but it quickly faces the barrier of cell wall, which exerts a counter force on the protoplast discouraging further water uptake. At this stage, if osmotic gradient is sufficient, water will continue to enter the cell leading to the development of enormous hydrostatic turgour pressure, which will distend the wall to its elastic limits.

The protoplasts at this stage also release unidentified 'wall loosening factors' which alter the wall's mechanical properties and allow it to undergo a process called 'stress relaxation'.

During stress relaxation, reversible wall extension (caused when there is no stress relaxation) is converted to a permanent irreversible wall extension, dramatically reducing both the wall stress and the turgour pressure. Thus, the plant cell expansion involves a continuous cycle of biochemical stress relaxation followed by turgour driven elastic extension. The stress relaxation is a biochemical event, while cell expansion is caused by passive water uptake. The cell expansion is also facilitated by a new class of cell wall proteins, called 'expansins' (isolated from cucumber and oats) which may play a key role in wall-loosening leading to cell expansion.

Cell Wall Loosening by Expansins: In 1992, a class of proteins, called 'expansins' (29kD) were identified, which induce expansion of growing cell walls, without any change in cell wall structure, although expansion of cell wall can also be caused by changes in its structure. This cell expansion property is particularly evident at an acidic pH (below), since expansins have an acidic pH optimum for induction of cell wall extension. Mature cells lack this acid induced cell extension. Expansins can be of two types - α -expansins and β -expansins. The α -expansins have high activity in cells walls of dicots and monocot grasses and the β -expansins have a reverse situation. Zea ml, the group 1 allergen of maize pollen is the typical example of β -expansin, and is involved in pollen tube growth, where it helps in loosening stigma and style walls, thus facilitating pollen tube growth. Another role of expansins may be in fruit ripening and the growth of leaf primordia. The mechanism of action of expansin is not fully understood, but perhaps they act by non-enzymatically breaking hydrogen bonds between cellulose fibres and hemicelluloses.

Orientation of Microfibrils and Control of Cell Shape: Another function of the cell wall is to determine cell morphology through its control on the orientation of the depositing microfibrils (Fig.).

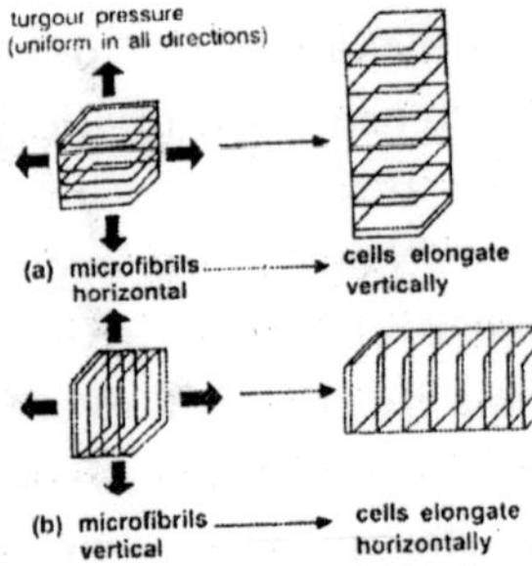

Influence of the orientation of cellulose microfibrils within the cell wall on the direction of cell elongation (redrawn from Alberts et. al., Molecular Biology of the Cell, 1994).

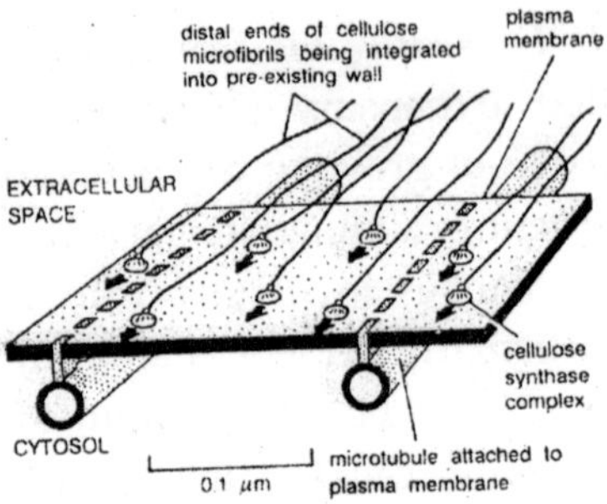

A model showing how the orientation of cortical microtubules determines the orientation of newly deposited cellulose microfibrils (redrawn from Alberts et. al., Molecular Biology of the Cell, 1994).

Cellulose is actually spun out from the outer surface of plasma membrane, with the help of cellulose synthase enzyme found in plasma membrane (Fig.). These cellulose molecules assemble into microfibrils and form a layer or lamella. All microfibrils have the same arrangement or alignment in a lamella. New lamellae keep on being formed internally to the previous ones, so that in a cell, lamellae are concentric and are perpendicular to the axis of cell elongation. On the inner side of plasma membrane are microtubules whose orientation can also influence the orientation of cellulose microfibrils, in the same fashion as the banks of a river or a canal direct the movement of water parallel to its banks. (Fig.). The mechanism involved in the regulation of the orientation of microtubules themselves is not fully understood.

Extracellular Matrix (ECM) in Animal Cells: Extracellular matrices (ECMs) in animal cells are insoluble networks found on the exterior of these cells and consist of macromolecules (proteins and polysaccharides) secreted by the cells into their immediate environment. In vertebrates, ECM differs in the different major tissue types including nerve, muscle, blood, lymphoid, epithelial and connective tissues. Of these, connective tissue and epithelial tissue represent two extremes with respect to the abundance of extracellular matrix (ECM). ECM is plentiful and sparse in 'connective tissue', but scanty forming a thin mat (basal lamina) in 'epithelial tissue.'

The connective tissue is the major component of skin and bone and forms only a minor component of organs like brain and spinal cord. On the other hand, epithelial sheets line all cavities and free surfaces of the body. ECM also exhibits great variation in the composition of macromolecules. This variation in the different types of macromolecules found in an ECM and the variation in the way they are organised in ECM gives an amazing diversity in ECM's structure, so that the matrix can become rock-hard in bone and teeth or may be a transparent structure as in cornea. ECM was earlier believed to provide mere stability to physical structures of tissues. But now we know that it plays a much more active and complex role in regulating the behaviour of animal cells, which come in its contact. It influences development, migration, proliferation, shape and function of contacting cells. Depending upon the type of tissue and organs, ECMs play several roles during development.

These functions include the following: (i) ECM helps in separation of two adjacent groups of cells (cell sorting) and prevent any interactions between them; (ii) ECM may serve as the substrate upon which cells migrate; (iii) ECM may induce the differentiation of certain cell types. In an embryo, at the base of epithelium, (*i.e.*, at the junction of epithelial cells and mesenchymatous cells), is found the basement membrane. This consists of ECMs in the form of 'basal lamina' formed due to epithelial cells and 'reticular lamina' secreted by mesenchymatous cells.

Formation of Extracellular Matrix: Extracellularlly matrix is really made up of macromolecules produced locally by cells which are embedded in the ECM itself. The orientation of these ECM macromolecules is actually determined by the orientation of the components of cytoskeleton of these embedded cells giving birth to ECM. In most connective tissues, the ECM molecules are secreted by the fibroblasts or by other cells of fibroblast family including chondroblasts in cartilage and osteoblasts in the bone.

Most ECMs are made up of the following two main classes of extracellular macromolecules: (i) polysaccharide chains of the class glycosaminoglycans (GAGs), which are covalently linked to proteins in the form of proteoglycans (except in case of 'hyaluronan') and (ii) fibrous proteins of two main types—structural (*e.g.*, collagen and elastin) and adhesive (*e.g.*, fibronectin and laminin). Sometimes, these extracellular macromolecules are also classified as small glycoproteins (*e.g.*, collagen and proteoglycans) and large glycoproteins (*e.g.*, fibronectin, laminin and elastin/entactin) (Table). These molecules are found in a wide variety of shapes and sizes performing a variety of functions (Fig.). In case of connective tissues, glycosaminoglycans (GAGs) and proteoglycans are highly hydrated and form gel-like 'ground substance,' in which fibrous proteins facilitate rapid diffusion of nutrients, metabolites and hormones between the blood and the tissue cells; collagen provides strength and helps organise the ECM; elastin fibres give it resilience (elasticity) ; the adhesive proteins help cells attach to appropriate parts of ECM; *e.g.*, fibronectin promotes attachment of fibroblasts and various other cells to ECM in connective tissue, while laminin promotes attachment of epithelial cells to the basal lamina.

Main Constituents of Extracellular Matrix (ECM).

Major constituents	*Mesenchymal ECM (reticular lamina)*	*Epithelial ECM (basal lamina)*
1. Small glycoproteins		
(a) Collagens	Long thin molecules assemble to form fibrils (60-70nm in diameter) ; most common is type I; types II, III, V-XIII also occur; provide strength and stability to tissues	Collagen IV as major component of basal lamina; fibrils assemble into sheet like substratum
(b) Proteoglycans	Made up of glycosaminoglycans (repeating disaccharides) like hyaluronic acid (10^8 Da), which binds large amount of water; sulphated proteoglycans have a core protein to which chains of sulphated glycosaminoglycans are attached (see Table)	Hyaluronic acid and sulphated proteoglycans are present and facilitate the passage of secretory products through the lamina
2. Large glycoproteins	Fibronectin, chondronectin and tenascin are found and allow adhesions of cells to facilitate their migration	Laminin is the major component with sites for adhesion of the cell membrane; collagen IV and glycosaminoglycans; fibronectin, entactin, nitrogen and other adhesive glycoproteins are also found.

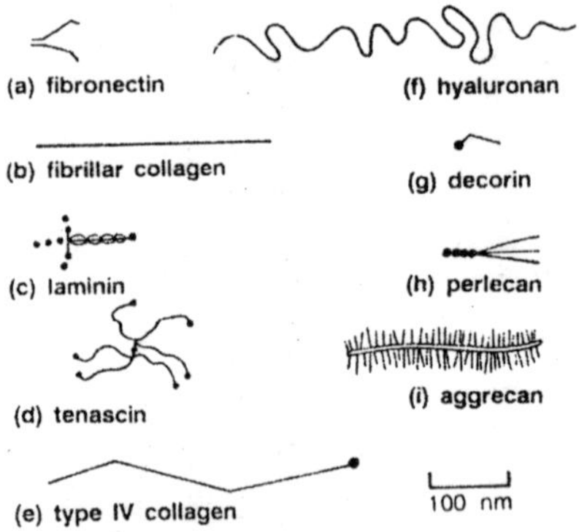

Comparative shapes and sizes of major macromolecules of extracellular matrix (ECM).

Glycosaminoglycans (GAGs) and Proteoglycans

Glycosaminoglycans (GAGs): GAGs in ECM are equal to only 10 per cent of the fibrous proteins by weight. They are unbranched polysaccharide chains consisting of disaccharide units (Table). One of the two sugar residues of a disaccharide unit, is often sulfated, having an amino group (N-acetylglucosamine or N-acetylgalactosamine), hence the name glycosaminoglycans (glycose is the general name for a monosaccharide and glycan is the general name for a polysaccharide). The second sugar is often a uronic acid (glucuronic or iduronic). Due to the presence of sulphate and carboxyl groups, GAGs are negatively charged.

Repeating Disaccharide Units of Most Common Glycosaminoglycans of ECM Protcoglycans.

Class of glyconsaminoglycans	*Repeating disaccharide unit*	*Location*
1. Hyaluronic acid	Glucuronic acid -N - acetylglucosamine	Connective tissue; bone, vitreous body of the eye
2. Sulphated glycosaminoglycans		

Contd...

Class of glyconsaminoglycans	*Repeating disaccharide unit*	*Location*
(a) Chondroitin sulphate	Glucuronic acid-N-acetylgalactosamine sulphate	Cartilage, cornea, arteries
(b) Dermatan sulphate	[Glucuronic or iduronic acid]—N- acetylgalacto-samine sulphate	Skin, heart, blood vessels
(c) Keratin sulphate	Galactose-N-acetylglu-cosamine sulphate	Cartilage, cornea
(d) Heparan sulphate	[Glucuronic or iduronic acid]—N-acetylgalact-osamine sulphate	Lung, arteries, cell surfaces

GAGs can not fold and take up globular shape; instead they remain highly extended, occupying huge volume relative to their mass (Fig.) and thus filling most of the extracellular space. They form gel even at low temperature and, due to negative charge, attract cations like Na^+ which are osmotically active, thus helping in sucking large quantities of water into the matrix. The ECM thus swells causing turgor to withstand forces. Due to this property of GAGs, the cartilage at our knee joints can withstand pressure of hundreds of atmospheres. The deficiency for a GAG can cause severe diseases. For instance a deficiency in the synthesis of 'dermatari sulphate' causes dwarfness, premature aging and generalised defects in skin, joints, muscles and bones.

Except hyaluronan, all GAGs are covalently linked to proteins giving rise to proteoglycans found in majority of animal cells (Fig.). 'Hyaluronan', itself is the simplest of the GAGs, consisting of 25,000 non-sulphated disaccharide units. It is found in all tissues and fluids in adult animals and is especially abundant in early embryos. Hyaluronan expands with water to occupy large volumes and therefore, is a space filler during embryonic development. It can be quickly and cheaply produced and, therefore, is also used in wound repair.

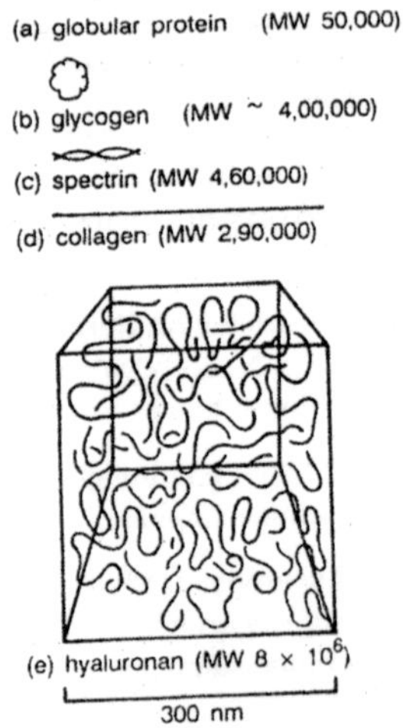

Volume occupied by hyaluronan, relative to its dimension (compare with that of other molecules).

Hyaluronan also helps in cell migration during formation of heart, cornea and other organs. After cell migration, excess hyaluronan is degraded by hyaluronidase enzyme. All the other GAGs occurring as proteoglycans have following common

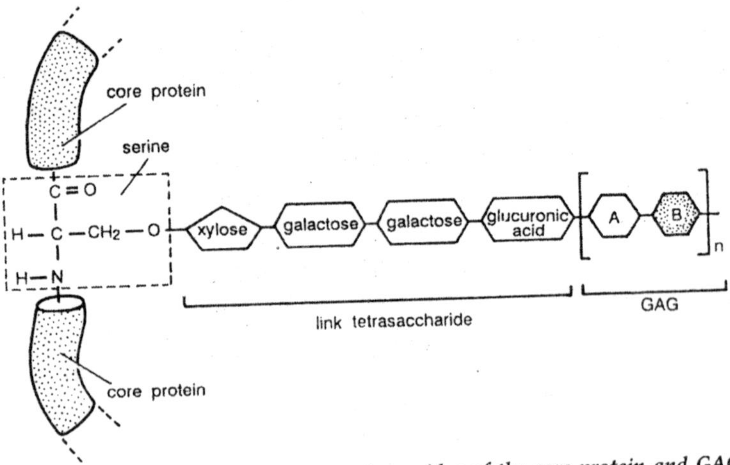

A tetrasaccharide linkage between serine residue of the core protein and GAG in a proteoglycan molecule (redrawn from Alberts et. al., Molecular Biology of the Cell, 1994).

features (i) they contain sulphated sugars; (ii) different disaccharide units are arranged in a complex manner in the same GAG; (iii) they are much shorter than hyaluronan, having fewer than 300 residues; (iv) they are covalently linked to proteins forming proteoglycans; (v) they are synthesized inside, the cell and released by exocytosis, while hyaluronan is spun out directly from the cell surface by an enzyme embedded in plasma membrane (as in case of cellulose for plant cell walls).

Proteoglycans. Proteoglycans (proteins + glycans, *i.e.* carbohydrates) are specific types of glycoproteins, which are characterised by the presence of carbohydrate component, which far exceeds the protein content and consists of linear chains of repeating disaccharide units. Usually one of the sugars of a disaccharide monomer has an amino group, so that the polysaccharide with this repeating unit is called a glycosaminoglycan (Table). The interconnections of protein and carbohydrate components lead to the formation of a web-like matrix. Following are some functions of proteoglycans:

(i) In many motile cell types, the proteoglycan surrounds the cells and prohibit the cells from coming together,

(ii) Proteoglycans also mediate connections between adjacent tissues of an organ. For instance, heparan sulphate (a glycosaminoglycan; see Table) proteoglycans bring together chondrocytes, the cartilage producing cells,

(iii) In still other cells, proteoglycans secreted by one cell type are essential for the growth of neighbouring cells, so that if proteoglycans (heparan sulphate) are removed from the surface, of axons of the dorsal root ganglia, the neighbouring Shwann cells do not proliferate,

(iv) Proteoglycans also help in binding of growth factors to their corresponding cell receptors. Details of some of the important proteoglycans are given in Table .

Some Common Proteoglycans

Proteoglycan and its location	*GAG chain (no. of chains)*	*Function*
1. Aggrecan (210,000)- cartilage	Chondroitin sulphate + keratin sulphate (-130)	Mechanical support
2. Beia-glycan (36,000) - cell surface-t-matrix	Chondroitin sulphate/ dermatan sulphate (1)	Binds TGF-0
3. Decorin (40,000) - connective tissue	Chondroitin sulphate / dermatan sulphate (1)	Binds TGF-/3
4. Perlecan (600.000)- basal laminae	Heparan sulphate (2-15) (basal lamina)	Structural & filtering
5. Serglycin (20,000) - secretory vesicles (WBC)	Chondroitin sulphate/ dermatin sulphate (10-15)	Packaging and storage of secretory molecule
6. Syndecan-1 (32,000) - fibroblast and epithelium	Chondroitin sulphate+ heparan sulphate (1-3)	Cell adhesion; binds FGF

*molecular weight of core protein in parentheses

The ratio of proteoglycans to collagen determines the consistency of ECM. Cartilage with high percentage of proteoglycans is soft; tendons which are predominantly collagen fibres are tough and the basal lamina having predominance of proteoglycans give structural support in addition to their function as molecular sieves.

Fibrous Structural Proteins

Collagens: Collagens are the abundant proteins (25 per cent of total protein mass) in mammals, found as a major component of skin and bone. They are glycoproteins, which are characterised as long, stiff, triple stranded structures, each strand being a collagen polypeptide chain called α -chain. The three strands are wound around one another in a superhelix. These collagen molecules are assembled into collagen fibrils, 10-300 μ m in diameter and hundreds of micrometers (μ m) long in mature tissues. These collagen fibrils may further aggregate into larger cable like bundles, described as collagen fibres (0.5-3nm in diameter). The molecules

(α helices) within a triple helix are cross-linked and the different triple helices are also cross-linked to each other due to intra- and inter-molecular cross-links (Fig.).

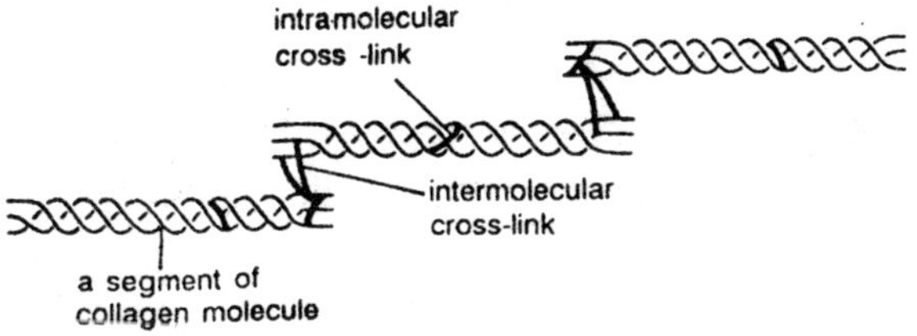

Intramolecular and intermolecular cross-links within a collagen fibril (redrawn from Alberts et. al., Molecular Biology of the Cell, 1994).

The above triple-helical (coiled-coil) structure for collagen was developed using x-ray diffraction patterns and was published for the first time in 1954 by the famous scientist Professor G.N. Ramachandran and his colleagues, then at the Physics Department of the University of Madras, (now it is the Department of Crystallography and Biophysics).

A closely related triple-helical structure for collagen was also proposed in 1955 by Alexander Rich and Francis Crick in Cambridge (UK) and by PM Cowan and collaborators at Kings College, London. Later this work on collagen led to an analysis of the general principles of folding of a polypeptide chain leading to the development of Ramachandran plot, which is most widely used now for the analysis of secondary and tertiary structures of proteins. The discovery of the triple-helix structure of collagen by Ramachandran has been considered to be as important, as the discovery of double helix structure of DNA by Watson and Crick in 1953. But the discovery of triple-helix model of collagen did not receive the same attention as the double helix model of DNA did, because DNA was considered far more important as the genetic material, although collagen is also, in its own right, the most abundant protein in mammals (one third of the protein in our own body is collagen).

Collagens are also characterised as glycoproteins which

are extremely rich in proline and glycine, both of which help in the formation of triple-stranded helix. Glycine (the smallest amino acid) is found at every third position in the central region of chain and prolinei due to its ring structure, stabilises the helical structure.

The collagen fibrils form structures that resist tensile forces, unlike GAGs which resist compressive forces. The collagen fibrils are, therefore, organised in different ways in different tissues: (i) In mammalian skin, they are interwoven in wickerwork pattern (pattern of twigs used in baskets, chairs, mats, etc.) so that tensile stress in many directions is resisted, (ii) In tendons, they are arranged in parallel bundles aligned along a major axis of tension, (iii) In mature bone and cornea, they are arranged in orderly plywood like layers, with fibrils in each layer parallel to each other but at right angle to those in the layer on either side.

In animal tissues 15 different types of collagen molecules, involving 25 different types of a chains are known. The main collagen types found in skin and bone are type I, II, III, IV, V and IX. Type I is the most common and particularly abundant in skin and bone. Some of the important collagens found in ECM, along with their characteristic features, functions and location are given in Table.

Collagen polypeptide α chains are synthesized on rough ER and are released as pro-α chains which not only have an amino-terminal signal peptide to direct the polypeptide to ER, but also have propeptides on both its ends. In ER lumen, selected proline and lysine residues are hydroxylated to form hydroxyproline and hydroxylysine respectively.

Three pro-α chains combine to form triple helical molecule called pro-collagen, which changes to collagen by removal of pro-peptides at the two ends. The collagen molecules first assemble in collagen fibrils (10-300nm) and then into collagen fibres (0.5-3mm) In scurvy (a disease caused by deficiency of vitamin C), the defective pro-chains fail to form a stable triple helix, and are therefore degraded within the cell.

Structural and Functional Heterogeneity of Major Classes (I-IV) of Collagens; other Classes (V-XHI) not Included

Collagen type (molecular formula)	*Characteristics and functions*	*Location*
Type I [α 1 (1)2 α 2(l)]	Low carbohydrate content; thick banded fibrils (bands 67nm wide) ; most abundant (makes 90% of total collagen in the body); gives high tensile strength	Skin, bone, tendon, ligaments, cornea
Type II [α 1 (II)],	High carbohydrate content; secreted by cartilage cells ; small banded fibrils (bands 67nm wide) forming compressible elastic matrix	Cartilage, notochord, vitreous body of the eye, intervertebral disc.
Type 111 [α 1 (III)]-,	High carbohydrate content ; triple helical; interchain disulphide bonds; small banded fibrils (bands 67nm wide) to provide support and elasticity	Skin, most evident in blood vessels; internal organs (excluding bone or tendon)
Type IV [α l(IV), α 2	'Chicken wire'-like fibrils; act as a cell attachment site and as a selective barrier; binds to laminin.	Basal laminae of ECM

Elastin: Elastin is a highly hydrophobia protein (about 750 amino acids), which is also proline and glycine rich (like collagen) but is not glycosylated. It contains little hydroxyproline and no hydroxylysine. The elastin protein is composed of (i) hydrophobic segments and (ii) alanine and lysine rich helical segments, the former providing elasticity and the latter forming cross-links between adjacent molecules.

These two types of segments alternate along the length of polypeptide chain. Elastin protein makes the elastic fibres, to which integrity is provided by another protein fibrillin. Mutation in fibrillin leads to Marfan's syndrome disease, where aorta (whose wall is rich in elastin) is prone to rupture.

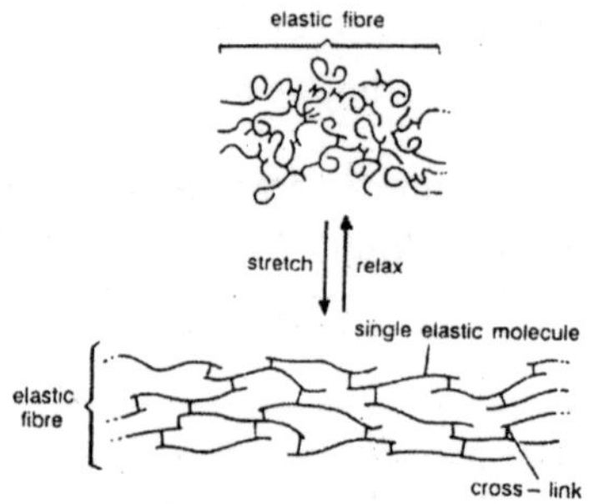

Expansion and contraction of elastin molecules joined together by covalent bonds (redrawn from Alberts et. al., Molecular Biology of the Cell. 1994).

Elastic molecules are secreted into the extracellular space and assemble into elastic fibres close to the plasma membrane. After secretion, elastin molecules become cross-linked to generate an extensive network of elastic fibres and sheets which are very common in tissues like skin, blood vessels and lungs. The elastic fibres are atleast five times more extensible than rubber band of the same thickness. In elastic tissues, collagen fibres are interwoven with elastic fibres to limit the extent of stretching, so that the tissue may not tear apart. The stretching and relaxation of elastin molecules is shown in Figure.

Fibrous Adhesive Proteins: ECM contains a variety of other specialised large glycoproteins (*e.g.* fibronectin, laminin, and tenascin), which are involved in arranging cells into organised structures through their function as substrate adhesive molecules. In the ECM, collagen and proteoglycan function as substrates, which utilise other substrate adhesive molecules for linking cells. These substrate adhesive molecules are also utilised for migration of one cell type on another cell type both having these substrate adhesive molecules on their surface as components of ECM. The substrate adhesive molecules also provide sites for attachment of colonising microorganisms.

Fibronectin: Fibronectin is a very large (460kD) glycoprotein dimer synthesized by cells like fibroblasts, chondrocytes, endothelial cells, macrophages and certain epithelial cells (*e.g.* hepatocytes and aminocytes). Two large subunits of a dimer fibronectin are joined by two disulphide bonds near their carboxyl termini (Fig.). Each subunit has a number of domains and each domain consists of smaller modules each of which is serially repeated. One of these modules is 'type III fibronectin repeat', about 90 amino acids in length. Fibronectin is a general substrate adhesion molecule and has binding sites (Fig.), whose interaction with appropriate molecules results in the proper alignment of cells with the ECM.

Fibronectin also helps in cell migration by making roads on which certain migrating cells travel, as illustrated by the following examples: (i) During gastrulation, certain mesodermal cells migrate on fibronectin surfaces of other cells and cease to migrate when fibronectin is removed, (ii) In chick embryos, the precursors of heart, *i.e.* the pre-cardiac cells migrate on fibronectin to travel from lateral side to the midline, so that if fibronectin is blocked (due to injection of antibodies, which will occupy the binding sites of fibronectin), migration will not take place and two hearts will develop.

Laminin: Laminin is a major component of basal lamina (see later for details) and provides a link between the cells and the structural components of basement membrane (found between epithelial and mesenchymatous cells). It is a large multi-chain glycoprotein and consists of three polypeptide chains, -A (440kD), B, (200kD) and B_2 (220kD).

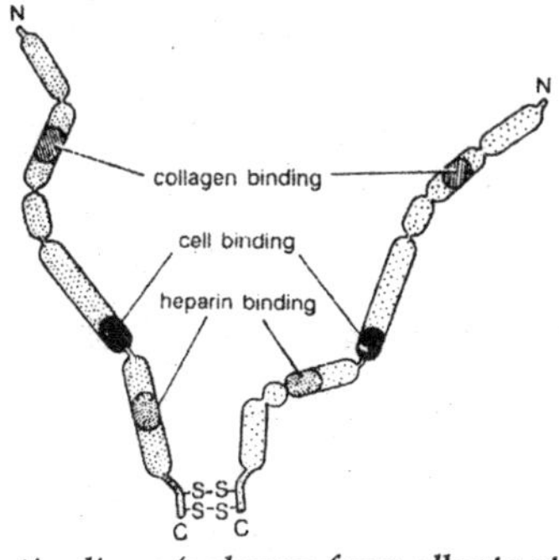

Structure of a fibronectin dimer (redrawn from alberts et. al., molecular Biology of the cell, 1994)

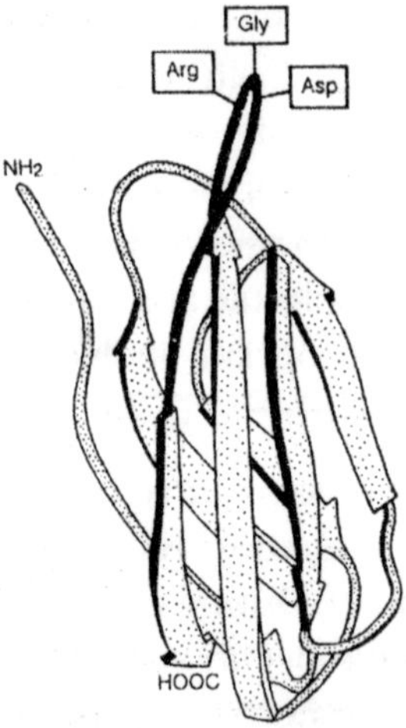

Three dimensional structure of type III fibronectin repeat, showing the major cell binding site in the form of Arg-Gly-Asp. (redrawn from Alberts et. al., Molecular Biology of the Cell. 1994).

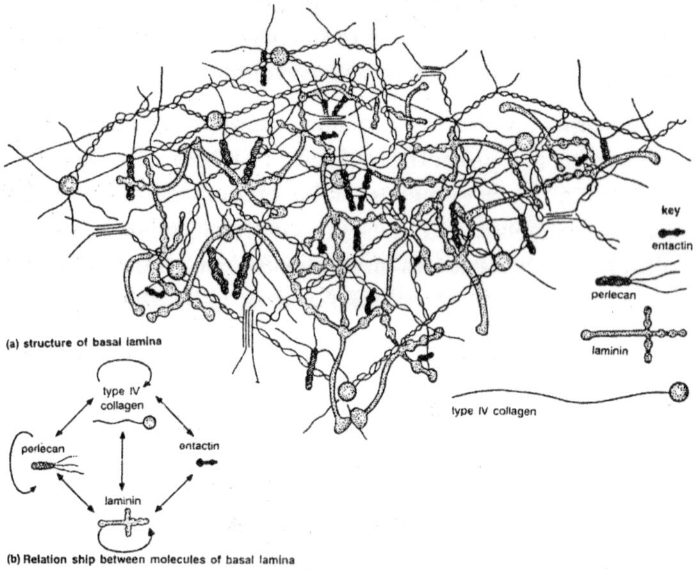

(a) A model of the structure of basal lamina organisation of different proteins (IV collagen, laminin, entactin, perlecan); Arrow connect molecules that can bind to each other. (redrawn from Alberts et. al., 'Molecular Biology of the Cell'. 1994).

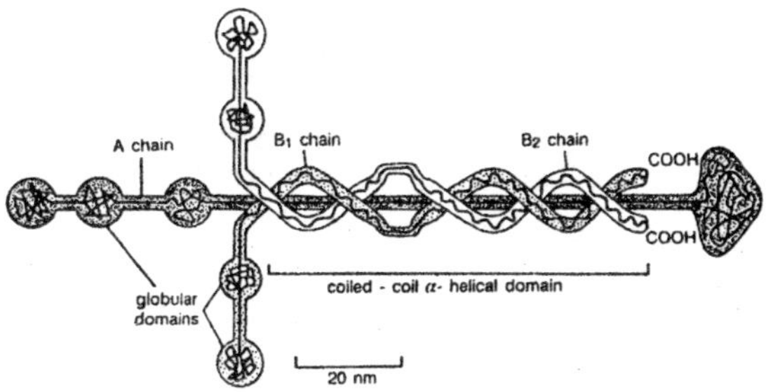

The structure of laminin, showing three polypeptides (A, B1, B2) that are cross-linked. (redrawn from Alberts et. al., 'Molecular Biology of the Cell', 1994).

These three polypeptide chains are repeated, but exhibit diversity in different organisms. The three chains are also linked via disulphide bonds to form an asymmetric cross structure (Fig.). Each of these three chains of laminin, have a number of functional domains, responsible for binding separately to type IV collagen, heparan sulfate, entactin and laminin receptors. A single dumb-bell shaped entactin molecule also binds to each laminin molecule. Entactin also binds to type IV collagen thus acting as a bridge between type IV collagen and laminin in the basal lamina (Fig.). Laminin has been isolated from a variety of organisms including mouse and fruitfly and its genes cloned and sequenced.

Laminin is the first ECM protein to appear during development. It is known to influence cell attachment, movement, differentiation and growth with the help of several laminin receptors, which have been identified as a class of cell surface receptors. Integrins and glycosyltransferases are two classes of such receptors. Laminin also binds to collagen (type IV) and glycosaminoglycans on the adjoining cells, thus functioning as a substrate adhesive molecule. The adhesion of epithelial cells to laminin is much greater than the affinity of mesenchymatous cells for fibronectin, since in the former case the cells sit and utilise the laminin for movement, while in the latter the mesenchymatous cells bind and release the laminin to help migration of mesenchyma over epithelium.

Tenascin (also called cytotactin). Tenascin resembles fibronectin for about half its length and is transiently found in several ECMs during embryonic development. However, different cells react differently to tenascin, so that it does not always promote cell adhesion.

Basal Lamina and ECM: At the interface between all epithelial cell sheets and connective tissues the matrix is organised as a thin but tough mat that is known as basal lamina. Basal lamina also surrounds individual muscle cells, fat cells and Schwann cells, which are separated from the underlying or surrounding connective tissue with the help of this basal lamina.

In kidney glomerulus and lung alveolus also, a basal lamina lies between two cell sheets and functions there as a highly selective filter. Basal lamina influences cell behaviour in a variety of ways. It determines cell polarity, influences cell metabolism and organises proteins in adjacent plasma membrane. Basal lamina also induces cell differentiation and serves as specific highways for cell migration.

The basal lamina strikingly differs from other examples of ECMs which mainly fill up the space between cells (*e.g.* connective tissue). The connective tissue itself also consists mainly of ECM, but basal lamina depends on some specialised types of ECM molecules including type IV collagen molecules which have more flexible structure than the collagen found in collagen fibrils.

They differ even in their biogenesis, because during synthesis, terminal regions, which hinder side to side packing, are not cleaved, but are retained for interaction to give a flexible sheet like multilayered network. These molecules make head to head dimers at carboxy-termini, which then arrange into an extended lattice via amino-terminal and other lateral associations (Fig.). These associations are stabilised by disulphide and other covalent cross-links.

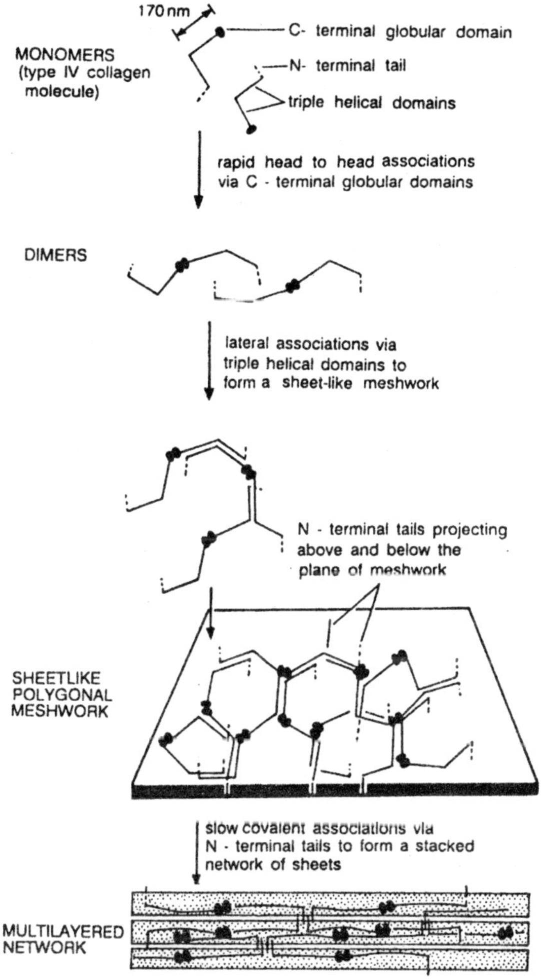

Different steps in the assembly of type IV collagen molecules into a inultilayered network (redrawn from Alberts et. al., 'Molecular Biology of the Cell', 1994).

Most basal laminae consist of two distinct layers (i) lamina lucida or rare lying towards, plasma membrane of say epithelial cells and (ii) lamina densa lying just below the lamina lucida. Sometimes a third layer (lamina fibroreticularis) is also found, which connects the basal lamina with underlying connective tissue. These three layers together, are sometimes also described as basement membrane, a term which has been used interchangeably for basal lamina.

The precise composition of basal lamina differs in different tissues or even in different regions of the same tissue, but the most important components of all basal laminae include type IV collagen, 'perlecan' (a heparan), laminin and entactin (large glycoproteins). As discussed earlier, laminin is the first ECM protein synthesized in developing embryo, when very little or no type IV collagen is found in ECM.

As earlier pointed out, basal lamina performs diverse and complex functions including the following: (i) Filtration of macromolecules in kidney glomerulus prevents passage of macromolecules from blood into urine and is facilitated by 'heparan sulphate' in basal lamina, so that if GAG chains of heparan sulphate are removed, the filtering properties of lamina are destroyed, (ii) A barrier provided by basal lamina does not allow fibroblasts from coming in contact of the epithelial cells, although macrophages, lymphocytes and nerve processes can pass through basal lamina, (iii) Wound repair, through regeneration, is facilitated by basal lamina, which provides a scaffold, along which regenerating cells can migrate to reconstruct the damaged tissue including muscle, nerve and epithelia Injuries in the nerve or the muscle at the neuromuscular junction (synapse) is also facilitated by the basal lamina, (iv) Cell migration during embryonic development is also regulated by basal lamina, so that mutation in a gene encoding components of basal lamina (*e.g.* laminin) disrupts the path of mesoderm cells or nerve axons that migrate over basal lamina (migration only along the dorsoventral axis is affected and that along the anteroposterior axis is not affected).

5

Role of Organelles

Cell Organelles

A eukaryotic cell is a complex structure and has a number of membrane bound compartments embedded in the cytoplasm. These compartments are called cell organelles. Of these intracellular compartments.

The other intracellular compartments include: (i) endoplasmic reticulum (ER), (ii) ribosomes, (iii) endosomes, (iv) Golgi complex, (v) lysosomes, (vi) hydrogenosomes (recently discovered) and (vii) centrosome. The relative volumes occupied by each of these organelles in a liver cell are shown in Table. Each of these compartments contains its own characteristic enzymes and other molecules, which are regularly transported from one compartment to another. Some of these molecules, in addition of serving as enzymes, also serve as organelle-specific surface markers, which direct the transport of proteins/lipids and other molecules to appropriate compartments. Each mammalian cell actually contains about 1 billion (10^9) molecules which can be classified into 10,000 kinds, which are mostly synthesized in the cytosol and then delivered to specific compartments. In this Chapter, we will describe these different intracellular compartments.

Relative Volumes Occupied by Major Intracellular Compartments in a Liver Cell.

	Intracellular compartment	*Relative volume (%)*	*Approx no./cell*
1.	Cytosol	54	1
2.	Mitochondria	22	1700
3.	Rough ER Cisternae	9	1
4.	Smooth ER cisternae + Golgi cisternae	6	—
5.	Nucleus	6	1
6.	Peroxisomes	1	400
7.	Lysosomes	1	300
8.	Hydrogenosome	< 1	—

Cytoplasmic Matrix (Cytosol): Cytoplasmic matrix or groundplasm, also described as cytosol, refers to the homogeneous plasma excluding all cell organelles visible under electron microscope. It is the most important part of the cell, which forms the true internal milieu. The cytoplasmic matrix is believed to be granular in structure, although it would be difficult to examine it outside the cell.

One of the important properties of matrix is its ability to undergo reversible sol-gel transformation which is attributed to colloidal properties of the cell. The colloidal property also helps in viscosity changes, intracellular motions (cyclosis), spindle formation and cell cleavage. Cytoplasmic matrix is also the site of many fibrillar differentiations such as microtubules and filaments. In the past, matrix was believed to consist of homogeneous peripheral part known as ectoplasm and the inner granular plasma known as endoplasm.

When the homogenised cells are subjected to cell fractionation, nuclear, mitochondrial and microsonial fractions are separated first. The remaining supernatant called soluble fraction or cytosol then contains the soluble proteins and enzymes found in matrix. These proteins and enzymes form 20-25 per cent of the total protein content of the cell. Several of these enzymes are either involved in glycolysis or in the activation of amino acids for protein synthesis. Soluble RNA (transfer RNA or t-RNA) is also found in this fraction.

A portion of cytoplasm which stains with basic dyes, is also called ergastoplasm (Gr., ergazomai-to elaborate and transform). This substance is primarily involved in biosynthesis. The basophilic property of ergastoplasm is known to be due to ribonucleic acid, since if the cell is treated with ribonuclease which destroys RNA, the staining property of ergastoplasm is lost. It is obvious thus that ergastoplasm is involved in protein synthesis. In the cytoplasmic matrix are also found the microtubules, microfilaments and intermediate filaments, which collectively constitute the cytoskeleton. Due to the significance, these structures have assumed in recent years.

Endoplasmic Reticulum (ER): In the cytoplasmic matrix described above, there is a vast network of closed and open cavities in the form of membrane bound tubules, vesicles and flattened sacs. This membranous organisation travelling the matrix is sometimes called cytoplasmic vesicular system, of which endoplasmic reticulum forms only a part. The other parts of this vesicular system are nuclear envelope, endosome, lysosome and Golgi complex.

Endoplasmic reticulum, generally abbreviated as ER, was previously unknown in the cytoplasm. Its presence in the cytoplasm is one of the most important discoveries made possible only through the use of electron microscopy. The name endoplasmic reticulum was used for the first time by K.R. Porter in 1948 to identify a fine-reticulum which he observed in the endoplasm of the cells.

Ultras Tructure: The strands of ER appear as a network of labyrinth consisting of branching tubules and flattened sacs with variable spaces. These strands form tubes and vesicles in the cytoplasm. Sometimes, there may be found chains of vesicles which are connected to one another by canalicules or large vesicles (Fig.). Obviously ER is a hollow system.

It is usually a continuous system, connected on one side to the nuclear envelope and on the other side to the cell membrane. However, in sectioned cells this continuity is not recognisable and the strands would appear as isolated circular or oval vesicles.

The ER membrane forms a continuous sheet enclosing a single internal space or a narrow lumen called ER lumen or ER cisternal space (Fig.). This narrow ER lumen is continuous into the lumen of the nuclear membrane so that ER system appears as an outgrowth of the nuclear membrane. The membrane of ER on its external surface carries granular structures known as ribosomes. The ER in certain regions may also be devoid of these ribosomes.

The ER regions carrying ribosomes are, therefore, called as rough endoplasmic reticulum and those devoid of ribosomes are known as smooth endoplasmic reticulum (Fig.).

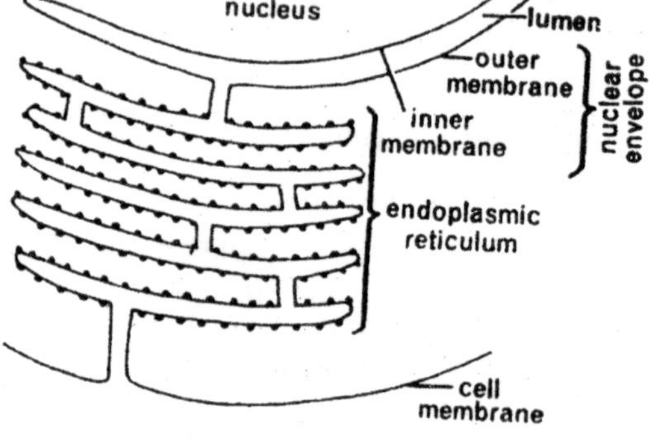

Endoplasmic reticulum as seen in section.

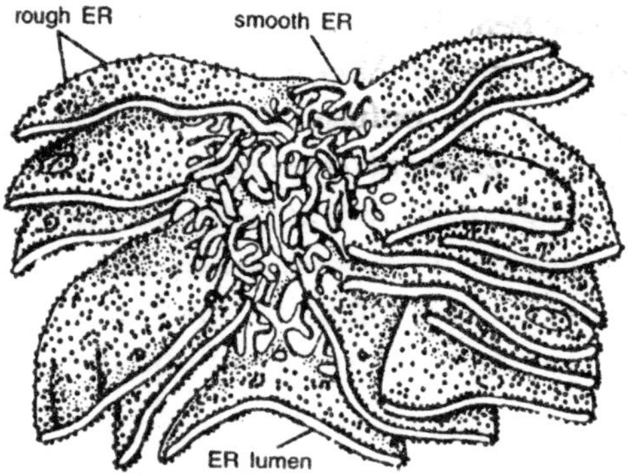

A three dimensional view of endoplasmic reticulum.

Rough Endoplasmic Reticulum (Granular): The rough endoplasmic reticulum is particularly well developed in cells actively engaged in protein synthesis. Generally it is found in that part of cytoplasm which is basophilic (ergastoplasm) a property which is attributed to attached ribosomes which contain RNA. Only rarely it has been found that a basophilic region is devoid of ER, since in these regions ribosomes are free. Such regions are found in embryonic animal and plant cells.

Rough endoplasmic reticulum is particularly well developed in pancreatic and liver cells where secretory proteins are synthesized on the attached ribosomes and are translocated through cisternae to different sites in the cells. The total surface of ER contained in 1 ml of liver tissue has been calculated to be 11 m^2, two third of which is rough ER.

Smooth Endoplasmic Reticulum (Agranular): Smooth ER forms a continuous system with rough ER, but has a different morphology. It consists of smooth membrane segments and found in regions rich in glycogen. Smooth ER is used for the formation of transport vesicles, which carry proteins and lipids to the Golgi complex.

Isolation and Chemical Composition: Microsomal fraction, as we know is obtained by differential centrifugation and consists of fragments of plasma membranes, rough and smooth ER and Golgi complex. Microsomes are no discrete entities, as sometimes these are confused with. If this microsomal fraction is subjected to gradient centrifugation, rough and smooth endoplasmic reticula as well as Golgi complex can be separated from one another. Moreover, when microsomal fraction is treated with deoxycholate (a surface active agent), the membrane system is destroyed and ribosomes can be isolated.

Endoplasmic reticulum has a high lipid content. There is more lipid relative to proteins in the smooth endoplasmic reticulum than in the rough endoplasmic reticulum. The latter also contains less sphingomyelin and cholesterol. The membrane proteins of ER have also been studied by polyacrylamide gel electrophoresis (a technique for separation of different proteins from one another in an electric field. As many as 30 polypeptide bands representing proteins ranging in molecular weight from 15,000 to 150,000 daltons could be identified in the rough ER.

Import of Proteins into ER (ER Signal Peptide, Signal Recognition Particle (SRP) and SRP Receptor): The ER network serves as a factory for the production of all lipids for the cell. Cytosolic surface is used for synthesis of majority of proteins. Further, all proteins synthesized in the cytosol and meant either for secretion or those destined for different cell organelles (ER, Golgi apparatus, lysosomes, the endosomes, etc.) and the plasma membrane are first imported into the ER lumen from the cytosol. In the ER lumen, these proteins fold and oligomerise (oligomerise means two or more polypeptides join together), the disulphide bonds are formed and N-linked oligosaccharides are added to form glycoproteins (N= asparagine).

The proteins which are imported into the ER lumen always carry a special hydrophobic signal peptide which facilitates their transport. This signal peptide is recognised by a signal recognition particle (SRP) which binds not only the growing polypeptide chain, but also the ribosome involved in the synthesis of this polypeptide chain. After binding, SRP directs the ribosome, along with the growing polypeptide chain to a SRP receptor located on the cytosolic surface of the membrane of rough ER. This initiates the process of translocation during which a loop of growing polypeptide chain traverses the ER membrane through a hydrophilic pore in a protein translocator

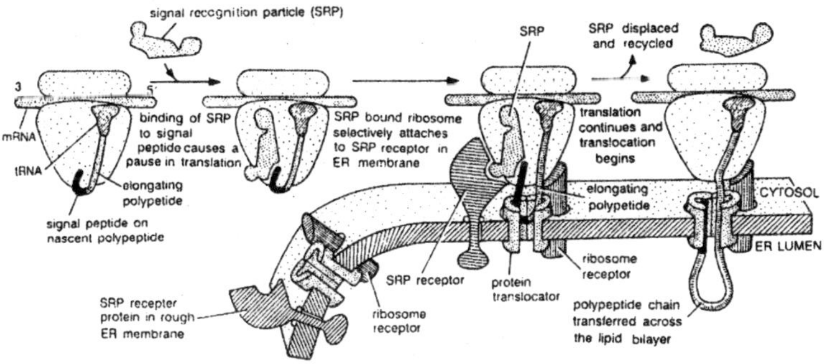

The role of ER signal peptide, SRP and SRP receptor in directing ribosome to ER membrane, (redrawn from Alberts et al., Molecular Biology of the Cell, 1994)

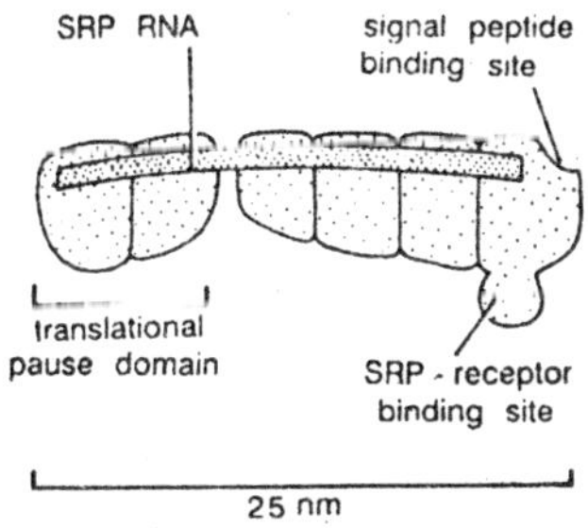

Structure of signal recognition particle (SRP) consisting of six protein subunits and one molecule of SRP RNA. (redrawn from Alberts et al., Molecular Biology of the Cell, 1994).

(see Fig. the membrane itself is hydrophobic, but the pore in protein translocator is hydrophilic). SRP itself is an elongated complex containing six protein subunits and one RNA molecule called SRP-RNA (Fig.). One end of this SRP binds to the ER signal peptide found in the growing polypeptide chain and the other end binds to the ribosome itself, stopping the translation temporarily. The SRP-RNA may interact with ribosomal RNA (rRNA). The SRP also has a site for the SRP receptor protein located on ER.

It is thus obvious that the import of proteins into ER is co-translational, while that into other organells (*e.g.* mitochondria, chloroplasts, nuclei peroxisomes, etc.) is post-translational. The proteins destined for ER are never released into the cytosol and no chaperonins are required to keep these proteins unfolded.

The proteins destined for ER can be of two types: (i) the soluble proteins which pass across the ER membrane and reach the ER lumen and (ii) the transmembrane proteins, which are destined for the ER membrane or other cell membrane, and therefore are not released in the lumen, but remain anchored in the lipid bilayer. This anchoring is facilitated by one or more α -helical regions (found in the polypeptide) spanning the membrane. These hydrophobic α -helical regions can function as start-transfer or stop-transfer signals during translocation. When several such α -helical regions acting as start/stop-transfer signals are found in a protein, it will pass back and forth across the membrane and form a multipass - transmembrane protein.

Functions: There are several possible functions, which endoplasmic reticulum performs. These functions include mechanical support, exchange and translocation of substances, protein synthesis, and the synthesis of lipoprotein and glycogen. These different functions will be briefly discussed.

Mechanical Support: Endoplasmic reticulum forms a network in cytoplasmic matrix and thus divides it into a number of chambers giving it the structure of a vacuolar system. In other words ER makes a part of the skeleton of the cell.

Exchange and Translocation: The fact that the endoplasmic reticulum forms $11m^2/ml$ of liver cells is an indication of enormous surface area which ER provides for exchange. Diffusion as well as active transport may regularly take place through the membrane system. The presence of carriers and permeases has been postulated to help ER membrane system to perform its function.

Endoplasmic reticulum may also act as a kind of circulatory system for intracellular circulation of various substances. It may help translocation of substances from the cytoplasm to outside the cell and *vice-versa*. For instance it helps to carry the raw materials to the site of cell wall formation. It also helps in the flow of RNA and the nucleoproteins from the nucleus to the cytoplasm which is the site of protein synthesis.

Protein Synthesis: Proteins are synthesized on the surface of rough ER. These proteins may be utilised within the cell or these may have to be exported outside the cell to the site of their utility. It is the latter kind of proteins in whose synthesis, endoplasmic reticulum plays an important role. For instance, rough endoplasmic reticulum, which has attached ribosomes, carries synthesis of secretory proteins on these ribosomes and export them. Synthesis of iropocollagen, serum proteins and secretion granules are some examples of secretory proteins. The protein molecules synthesized on attached ribosomes are discharged and penetrate into the cavity of ER, where they are either stored or exported outside. During the transport of these products, three types of membranes, ER- Golgi membrane - plasma membrane should interact and remain interconnected or disconnected due to membrane fusion and fission respectively.

Synthesis of Lipoprotein and Glycogen: As shown above, the rough ER, due to ribosomes, is engaged in protein synthesis. On the other hand smooth ER is engaged in synthesis of lipids in collaboration with Golgi complex. In the liver, the smooth ER is abundant in the hepatocytes and is involved in the production of lipoprotein particles, which carry the lipids to other parts of the body. The smooth ER is also known to be involved in the synthesis of glycogen as shown by their close association.

Detoxification of Drugs: The membrane of smooth ER, besides containing the enzymes for lipid synthesis also contains enzymes that detoxify lipid soluble (but water insoluble) drugs and other harmful compounds. Cytochrome P450 family is one important example of detoxification enzymes, which render these drugs water soluble, so that these may leave the cell and are excreted in the urine. When large quantitites of these harmful compounds enter the circulation, detoxification enzymes are synthesized in large quantities and smooth ER doubles its surface area within a few days. Once these harmful compounds are detoxified and removed, the excess smooth ER is removed by lysosome-dependent autophagocytosis.

Release, uptake and Storage of Ca^{2+}: The ER also releases Ca^{2+} into the cytosol and reuptake it. This release and uptake of Ca^{2+} helps in rapid responses to extracellular signals. The storage of Ca^{2+} in ER lumen is facilitated by presence of Ca^{2+} binding proteins there. In muscle cells, specialized ER, called sarcoplasmic reticulum (SR) sequesters Ca^{2+} from the cytosol using Ca^{2+}-ATPase pumps. The release and uptake of Ca^{2+} by SR helps in muscle contraction.

RNA Localisation in Oocyte: The vegetal end of the oocyte often contains RNAs that may control germ cell specification and axial pattern in the developing embryo. It was shown recently (in 1997) that the translocation of some of these mRNA molecules (*e.g.* Vgl mRNA in *Xenopus*) is brought about by a subdomain of the endoplasmic reticulum.

Origin: The origin of endoplasmic reticulum is not definitely known. One hypothesis assumes that it may develop as an evagination from the nuclear envelope. At telophase, the nuclear envelope is reformed with the help of vesicles of ER. In order to understand relationship of rough ER and smooth ER, so far as their origin is concerned, differentiating cells were studied. While in early stages rough ER is more abundant, subsequently smooth ER increases in quantity. Incorporation of radioactive amino acids into lipoproteins also suggested that the synthesis of membranes follows the direction, rough ER to smooth ER.

Ribosomes: Ribosomes are cell organelles, which function as cell's protein factories. They provide for the sites of protein synthesis involving translation of the genetic information encoded in the messenger RNA (mRNA). When not engaged in protein synthesis, the ribosomes in a prokaroytic cell are always free, but in a eukaryotic cell, these may be found either free in the cytosol or attached on the ER (rough ER).

In bacteria like *E. coli*, an individual ribosome (sedimenting at 70S; ~2.5MD; MD = megadelton) has an average diameter of 21-23nm (lnm = 10Å), and consists of two subunits, a smaller subunit (sedimenting at 30S) and a larger subunit (sedimenting at 50S). The ribosomes that are found in plastids and mitochondria largely resemble those in bacteria, although there are some variations. In eukaryotes, on the other hand, the ribosome is slightly bigger in size (80S;.~4.2MD), consisting of 40S smaller and 60S larger subunit (Table). The association of the subunits into a complete ribosome is facilitated by Mg^{++} ion concentration, so that at a specific lower Mg^{++} ion concentration, the subunits fall apart and at sufficiently higher Mg^{++} ion concentration, the ribosomes may form dimers. When engaged in protein synthesis, ribosomes can be found in clusters as polyribosomes, held together with the help of mRNA.

Ultrastructure: The structure of the two subunits and that of the complete bacterial ribosome as viewed under the electron microscope is shown in Figure. It can be seen that the smaller subunit consists of a head, a base and a platform, the platform separating the head from the base with the help of a cleft (also called shoulder). The larger subunit seems to be a solid monolithic structure having a ridge a central protuberance (CP) and a stalk, the ridge and CP separated by a valley.

Classes of Ribosomes and their Subunits.

Source of ribosomes	*Sedimentation coefficient (whole ribosome & the 2 subunits)*	*Sedimentation coefficient of ribsomal ribosomal RNA (rRNA)*
Liver, Yeast, Bean, *Neurospora*	80S (60S, 40S)	28S, 18S
E. Coli, Chloroplasts	*70S* (50S, 30S)	23S, 16S
Mitochondria	60S-78S	

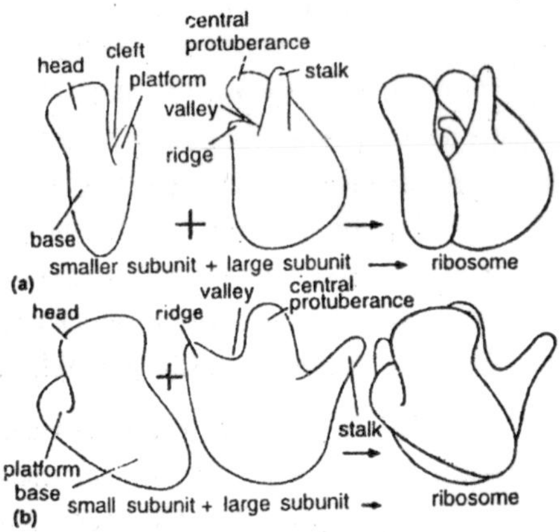

Three dimensional model of E.coli ribosome shown in two different orientations (A and B) (redrawn from Sci. Amer. Vol. 245. 1981).

Chemical Composition and Organisation: Each bacterial ribosome contains three species of ribosomal RNA (rRNA) and more that 50 different ribosmal proteins (r-proteins) (Fig.). The rRNA makes as much as 60-70 per cent of the ribosome. The 30S subunit is composed of 16S rRNA (-1500 nt; nt = nucleotides) and 21 different proteins (S1 to S21), whereas the 50S subunit contains 23S rRNA (-3000 nt), 5S rRNA (120 nt) and more than 30 different r-proteins (LI to L34). A similar organisation is also found in a eukaryotic ribosome, although in addition to the above, a 5.8S rRNA species is also found in eukaryotes (28S rRNA = -5000 nt; 18S rRNA = -2000 nt; 5.8S rRNA = 160 nt; 5S rRNA = 120 nt). It has been possible to dissociate rRNA and r-proteins from ribosomal subunits, and reconstitute the subunits from its components, so that if the reconstitution of ribosomes was allowed in the absence of a specific r-protein, the function of this protein could be studied. The location of some important proteins and sites for specific functions are shown in Figures.

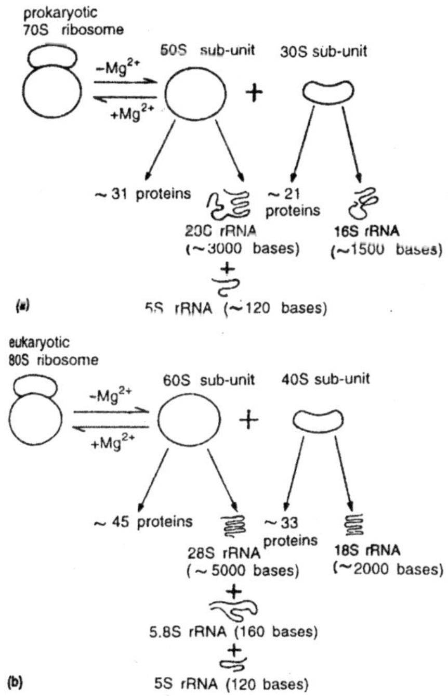

Different RNA and protein components of prokaryotic ribosomes (a) and eukaryotic ribosomes (b).

During 1970s and 1980s, details of structures of individual rRNA species and the different r-proteins were determined by X-ray crystallography and nuclear magnetic resonance (NMR) spectroscopy. The analysis of the structure of rRNA had suggested that due to intrastrand complementarity among the nucleotides of the same rRNA species, there are extensive double stranded regions in the different species of rRNA found in a ribosome.

The different regions of individual rRNA species including the double stranded regions were also classified in structural domains. The 16S rRNA has four such structural domains (5' domain, central domain, 3' domain and 3' minor domain), while 23S rRNA and the associated 5S rRNA together have six such domains (I-VI).

There are also a number, of helical stems in each rRNA, which are serially numbered, strarting from the 5' end : ~50 helices in 16S rRNA (H1-H45; some of the numbers are used with subscripts a, b, etc. for more than one stem), and > 100 in 23S rRNA. The double helical regions generally do not exceed 10 base pairs (bp), and these duplex regions are often imperfect having bulges of unpaired bases.

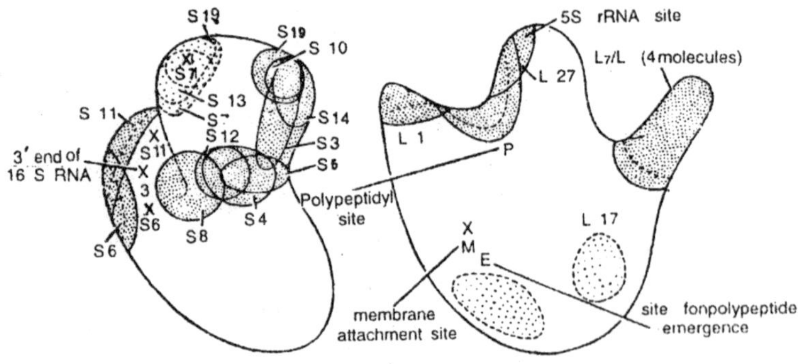

Map of proteins in the ribosome showing their position in small submit (left) and the large submit (right).

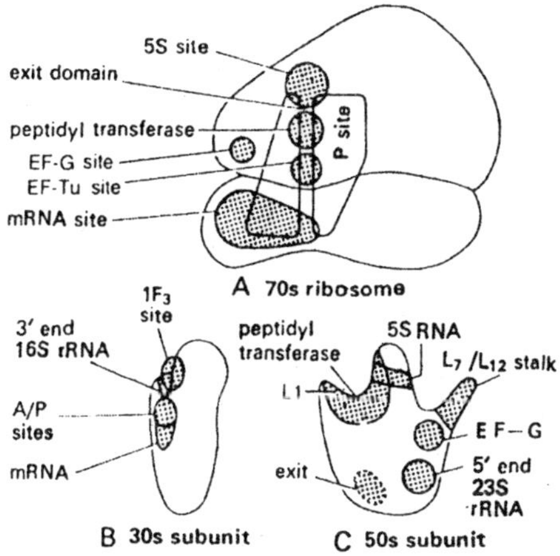

Some important centres (sites) for specific functions in the ribosome and its subunits.

The amino acid sequences and the three dimensional (3D) structures of most of the r-proteins were also available for some time. But complete information about the spatial distribution of rRNA species and >50 different proteins within ribosomal subunits, and the interactions between different regions of these macromolecules were determined only during 1999-2000.

High Resolution Structure (Atomic Level) of Ribosome Using Cryoelectron Microscopy (Cryo-EM) and X-ray Crystallography: During the last two decades (1980-2000) significant progress in the study of ribosome structure was achieved using the following two different approaches, (i) The first approach involved cyro-EM study which gave a resolution of upto , 8Å. This allowed a study of ribosome's surface topography, where all the cavities and bulges were resolved. The manner in which mRNA threads itself through the ribosome was also resolved by cryo-EM. (ii) The second approach involved X-ray crystallography of each of the two subunits (30S and 50S) at a resolution of 3Å and 2.4Å respectively, and of the entire bacterial ribosome (70S) at a resolution of 7.8Å.

The latest results of this work involving the preparation of electron density maps of ribosome and its subunits were published during 1999 and 2000 in a series of research papers. Three dimensional (3D) images of ribosome bound to mRNA and tRNA were also obtained, to study the interaction of ribosome with mRNA and tRNA.

The above studies allowed localisation of the positions of different domains of rRNA and those of a majority of ribosomal proteins belonging to the subunits. For instance, it was shown that the morphological features and the functionally important regions of ribosome and its subunits (*e.g.*, 30S-50S interface, and the active site of peptidyl transferase) are largely determined by the r-RNA component rather than by r-proteins. The r-proteins on the other hand are though dispersed throughout the structure, are mainly concentrated on its surface. This involves protein-rRNA interactions as well as protein-protein interactions which stabilise the organisation of different domains of rRNAs within the subunits.

In the 50S subunit of ribosome, the six domains of 23S rRNA and 5S rRNA, all have complex shapes, 'which fit together to produce a compact monolithic RNA mass in 50S subunit (Fig.). In contrast to this, in the 30S subunit, the 5′ domain of 16S rRNA makes bulk of the body, the central domain makes most of the platform, 3' major domain makes bulk of the head and the 3' minor domain makes part of the body at the 30S-50S interface. Thus the three major domains of 16S rRNA fit nicely in the three structural domains of 30S subunit. This difference between the two subunits in the organisation of their respective rRNAs may allow greater conformational flexibility for the smaller subunit.

Among the r-proteins, structure and organisation of all proteins except L10 have been resolved at the atomic level. The organisation of these proteins differ from that in the spherical viruses (proteins forming a shell) as well as from that in the eukaryotic nucleosomes (histones making a core with DNA wrapped on it). The 30S-50S interface is largely free of proteins except SI2, which lies near the decoding site. Within the ribosomal subunits, many loops and termini of these proteins were actually shown to penetrate between RNA helices, so that they are involved in stabilisation of the 3D structure of rRNAs, by functioning like 'mortar' or 'modelling clay,' filling the gaps and cracks between "RNA bricks".

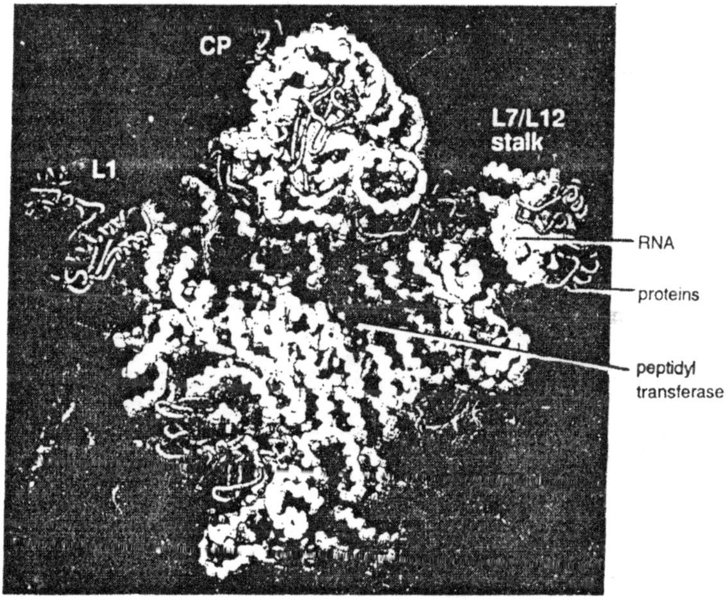

The high resolution compact monolithic structure of 50S subunit of E. coli ribosome, showing r-RNA and proteins.

Function (Ribosome as a Ribozyme-peptidyl Transferase): Ribosomes work as protein factories and provide for the sites of translation of the genetic information available in the form of mRNA. This function involves (i) acceptance of correct aminoacyl-t-RNA by decoding of m-RNA, (ii) peptide bond formation, (iii) translocation of peptidyl-tRNA from A site to P site, and that of deacylated t-RNA from P-site to E-site, and (iv) the exit of deacylated-t-RNA from the ribosome. The 30S subunit is involved in decoding, and in association with the 50S subunit, it is also involved in translocation; 50S subunit, on the other hand, functions as a ribozyme, helping in peptide bond formation.

A tRNA molecule can bind at any of the three sites available on the ribosome. These three sites include aminocacyl or acceptor site (A-site), peptidyl site (P-site) and the exit site (E-site). Each binding site is partitioned between the two ribosomal subunits, thus making six different sites of interaction between tRNA and the ribosome (Fig.). The anticodon end of tRNA binds to 30S subunit (which also carries mRNA), and its 3'-acceptor or CCA end interacts with the 50S subunit. The 50S subunit also contains the peptidyl transferase (a ribozyme), which is the catalytic site for peptide bond formation Thus the tRNA spans the interface between 30S and 50S subunits.

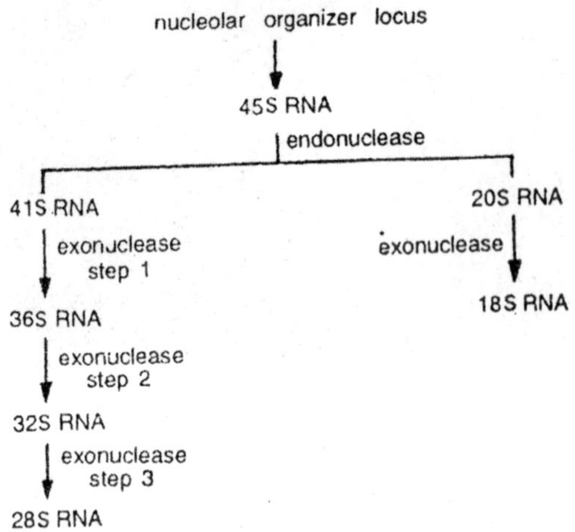

Schematic representation showing synthesis of 28S and 18S rRNA from nucleolar organiser loci.

Among the functions of ribosome listed above, elongation of peptide during translation is the most important and is the only enzymatic function. It involves selection of aminoacyl tRNA at the A site (decoding site), peptide bond formation between aminoacyl tRNA and the peptidyl tRNA and the translocation of newly formed peptidyl tRNA from A site to the P site. All these three steps are based on properties of ribosome itself (probably on rRNA), although in vivo AA-tRNA selection and translocation do need elongation factors EF-Tu and EF-G. Molecular mechanisms involved in the above functions of ribosome are still not completely understood and will be the subject of future research.

However, the most remarkable discovery during 1999-2000, was that ribosome was found to be a ribozyme. In this study it was shown unambiguously, that it is the 23S rRNA and not an r-protein, which works as a ribozyme and performs the function of peptidyl transferase for the formation of peptide bonds during elongation of polypeptide being synthesized.

Biogenesis: In bacteria, the genes for 5S, 23S and 16S rRNAs are clustered in one region to form a single operon working as a functional unit. In eukaryotes, however, the biogenesis of ribosomes is more complex involving several regions of the cell. The 18S, 5.8S and 28S rRNA molecules are synthesized as much bigger molecules in the nucleolar organiser which has multiple copies of ribosomal DNA repeat units responsible for the synthesis of rRNA In eukaryotic cells, initially rRNA is synthesized as a 45S precursor molecule, which later gives rise to 41S and 20S rRNAs due to enzymatic action (enzyme) endonuclease is utilised).

While 41S molecule forms 28S rRNA due to exonuclease action, 20S molecule gives rise to 18S molecule (Fig.). The DNA responsible for 5S rRNA is also repetitive (with many copies) but is synthesized outside the nucleolus. Formation of rRNA is coupled with formation of different ribosomal proteins which are synthesized in the cytoplasm. However, most of the subunits of ribosomes are processed in the nucleolus and delivered to the cytoplasm, suggesting a key role of nucleolus in the biogenesis of ribosomes.

Golgi Intricate

Golgi apparatus was described for the first time by C. Golgi (1822-1885) in nerve cells. Since originally these were known to be networks, they were also called dictyosomes (Greek, dictyes=net). a term that was later abandoned. 'Golgi complex' has been considered to be more appropriate.

The Golgi complex has a key position in the functioning of the membrane system of the cell. Besides performing synthetic functions, Golgi complex provides connection between ER and perinuclear space on the one hand and between transport vesicles and plasmalemma on the other. Since it provides connection with the nucleus, it also performs an important function for transport of material from the central control site (nucleus) to the cytoplasm.

Ultrastructure: The Golgi complex varies in form from a compact discrete granule or mass to a dispersed filamentous reticulum. The shape and function of this organelle varies with the metabolic state of the cell. In other words Golgi complex is pleomorphic. It consists of a series of double membranes, concentrically bent (Fig.) These double membranes are really flattened membrane-bound sacs, which are also referred to as cisternae', 'saccules' or 'lamellar units'.

These individual vesicles or sacs (60 nm in diameter) are sometimes also referred to as 'dictyosomes' or 'golgiosomes'. Size of these cisternae varies and their number in Golgi ranges from 3 to 12. Cisternae of lamellae are interconnected and stacked together forming Golgi stacks, each stack consisting of 4-6 cisternae. A large number of small vesicles that remain associated with each Golgi stack transport proteins and lipids, both to and from the Golgi apparatus. Each Golgi stack has two faces, a *cis* face (entry face, which receives vesicles from ER) and a *trans* face (exit face, from where Golgi vesicles leave the Golgi stack). Each of these faces *(cis* and *trans)* are closely connected to a network of interconnected tubules and thus from cis Golgi network (CGN) and trans-Golgi network (TGN).

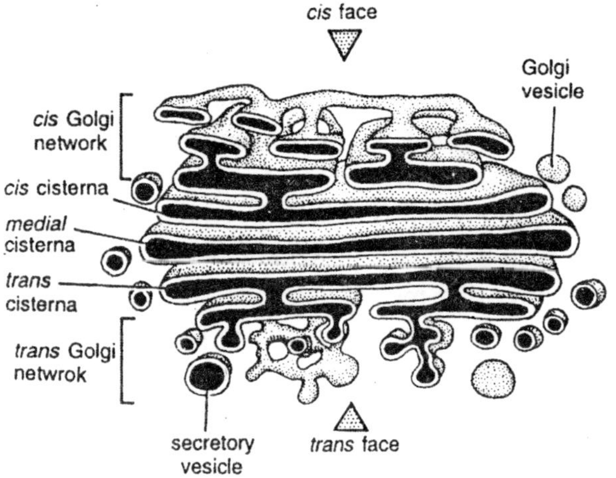

A three dimensional view of golgi complex.

Isolation and Chemical Compositioin: The isolation of Golgi complex is brought about mainly by gentle homogenisation followed by differential and gradient centrifugation. Gentle homogenisation allows preservation of stacks of cisternae. Since Golgi complex has a lower density than ER or mitochondria, it forms a distinct band in gradient centrifugation. Washing with distilled water leads to purification of Golgi complex, although its secretory components may be lost.

Golgi complex mainly consists of lipoproteins. In rat liver it consists of protein and lipids in a ratio 60 : 40. Some of the proteins are common with ER as shown by gel electrophoresis technique but on an average Golgi complex has fewer proteins which it receives perhaps from rough ER. Golgi complex also has very low level of RNA, DNA and polysaccharides. Although enzymes of plasma membrane, ER, mitochondria and peroxisomes are also found in Golgi complex, main enzymes are thiamine pyrophosphatase and glycosyl transferases.

Function: The Golgi complex is involved in the transport of macromolecules between the cells (intercellular level) or within the cell (intracellular level), a process often described as membrane trafficking.

For export the material is packaged into vesicles, which are detached and transported across plasmalemma, by a process of reverse pinocytosis or exocytosis. In animals, such material exported by Golgi complex, includes zymogen of pancreatic cells, mucous secretions, lactoprotein of mammary gland cells, compounds of thyroxin, melanin granules and other pigments, tropocollagen and collagen. Similarly, in plants the materials exported through Golgi complex include components of primary and secondary walls. Golgi complex is also involved in the formation of cell plate during cell division.

Another membrane trafficking event, extensively, studied in recent years, is the transport within the Golgi apparatus (intra-Golgi transport). This transport between Golgi cisternae involves the following steps: (i) the donor cisterna gives birth to a coated bud; (ii) the bud is detached and is targeted to acceptor cisterna; (iii) the bud is uncoated and attaches to acceptor cisterna; (iv) a 'fusion machine' (a complex of three proteins) assembles at the interface and helps in fusion of bud with the acceptor cisterna, thus depositing its contents.

Origin: The formation of Golgi complex may involve the synthesis of cisternae and there is variation in the number and size of cisternae in each stack.

This may be brought about in one of the following ways: (i) Individual stacks of cisternae may arise from pre-existing stacks by division or fragmentation. This will be little different than a *de novo* formation of apparatus, (ii) Cisternae membranes may arise from rough ER, which changes to smooth ER and eventually becomes the Golgi cisternae. Many cytological and biochemical studies lend support to this theory.

Endosome

Structure and Chemical Composition: Endosome (sometimes also called receptosome) is an organelle, that was discovered in recent years. It is a heterogenous structure consisting of membrane bound tubules and vesicles. It is involved in intracellular traffic and in sorting of ligands and receptors. It has been shown that the endosomes (like lysosomes) have an acidic medium with pH ranging from 5.0 to 5.5 (pH in lysosomes is generally 6.0).

This low pH is maintained through H^+ pumps. Endosomes have their origin through endocytosis. The coated vesicles resulting from endocytosis, get transformed into endosomes, while later become acidified. Endosomes are sometimes also considered to be the precursors of lysosomes and differ from them only in the absence of degradative enzymes and a slightly lower pH.

Types of Endosomes: There are at least two types of endosomes: (i) Early endosomes lie just beneath the plasma membrane and receive endocytosed proteins within about one minute, (ii) Late endosomes are closer to the nucleus and receive endocytosed proteins within 5-10 minutes. The early endosomes are actually involved in sorting proteins during endocytic pathway. The relationship between the above two types of endosomes and the lysosomes is not fully understood. However, it has been shown that early endosomes may mature into late endosomes, which in turn mature into lysosomes. The pathway is unidirectional, so that a protein leaving the early endosome for the late endosome, will end up in the lysosome.

Function: A ligand may enter the cell with or without a receptor. The ligands entering the cell without the help of a receptor, get fused with the lysosome. However, when a ligand enters the cell, in association with a receptor, the endosome may disallow its immediate fusion with the lysosome, so that this endosome gets time to sort out the ligand from its receptor. For instance, LDL (low-density lipoprotein particle a ligand) is endocytosed using an LDL receptor; the ligand finds its way to the lysosome and gets degraded, while the receptor due to the presence of a signal sequence, is recycled (not degraded) to the plasma membrane to be used again.

The rescue of the receptor is carried out in the endosome, where due to low pH, uncoupling of ligand and the receptor takes place. In another case (*i.e.* EGF or epidermal growth factor), both the ligand and the receptor are degraded in the lysosome. In still another case, transferrin (iron transporting protein), the receptor and the ligand both are rescued. Later the iron is separated from the transferrin and gets incorporated into the cytoplasm.

Lysosomes: As a result of electron microscopic studies, rounded dense bodies were observed in liver cells. These bodies were initially described as pericanalicular dense bodies. Such a term only suggested their location and not their function. In 1955, C. de Duve renamed these organelles as 'lysosomes', because they contain digestive enzymes capable of lysis. A lysosome, therefore, is a lytic body.

Structure and Occurrence: The lysosomes appear as dense bodies in the cell and are surrounded by a membrane. The interior contains a granulated stroma and a vacuole. Their shape and density vary greatly. These are 0.23 -0.50 μ in size. Due to variability in shape and size, their identification is rather difficult. The only criterion for their identification is the presence of lytic enzymes. Although the lysosomes are believed to be common in animal cells only, their general distribution in the animal cells suggested that they may be found in plant cells also. In 1964, P. Matile demonstrated the presence of lysosomes in *Neurospora*.

Isolation and Chemical Composition: Lysosomal fraction is isolated by centrifugation after mild homogenisation. The fraction usually has contamination of mitochondria and microsomes, but pure fractions of liver lysosomes have been obtained in good quantity.

However, considerable polymorphism shown by lysosomes in different cells and even within a single cell makes their identification rather difficult.

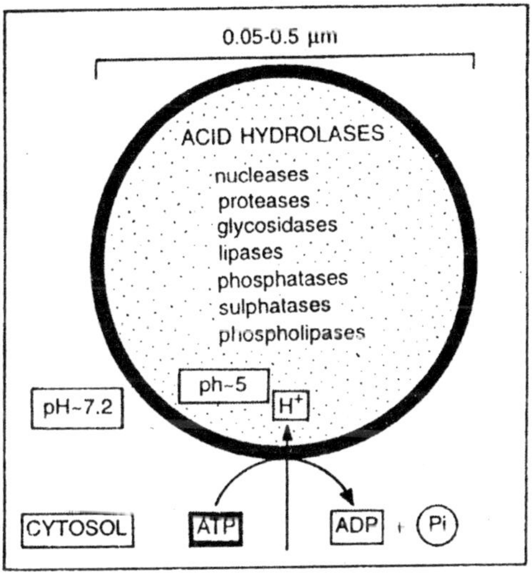

A lysosome containing a number of acid hydrolases, that are active under acidic condition, which is maintained by an H^+ ATPase in the membrane (redrawn from Alberts et al. Molecular Biology of the Cell, 1994)

Each lysosome contains about 40 types of hydrolytic enzymes (proteases, nucleases, glycosidases, lipases, phospholipases, phosphatases, sulphatases). For the activity of these acid hydrolases, the lysosomes maintain a pH of about 6 in its interior. If these enzymes leak into cytosol (pH =7.2), they can do little damage at higher pH there.

The lysosome membrane also contains transmembrane proteins, which help in transport of the final products of digestion to the cytosol, where they can be either excreted or reutilised by the cell. The lysosomal membrane also has H^+

pumps; which utilise the energy released due to ATP hydrolysis to pump H^+ into the lysosome, thus maintaining the lumen at its acidic pH of ~ 5 (Fig.). Most of these lysosomal membrane proteins are highly glycosylated, which perhaps protect them from lysosomal proteases.

Types of Lysosomes: Following types of lysosomes are recognised, depending upon the function they have to perform. Primary lysosome, also known as starch granule is a small body having enzymes synthesized by ribosomes attached to endoplasmic reticulum. These enzymes first enter the Golgi complex where an acid phosphatase reaction takes place, before they are transported to primary lysosomes which may be preferentially charged with one type of enzyme or another. The acid hydrolases are present only in secondary lysosomes. Using autoradiography technique, the transfer of protein was observed to have the following sequence: ER $\rightarrow$ Golgi complex $\rightarrow$ lysosomes.

Secondary lysosome, also known as heterophagosome or digestive vacuole, results from phagocytosis or pinocytosis of foreign material by the cell. It shows a positive phosphatase reaction, which may be due to association with primary lysosome. The engulfed material is digested by hydrolytic enzymes. The products of digestion pass through the membrane of lysosome and are incorporated into the cell.

Residual bodies are formed if the digestion is incomplete. These residual bodies are removed by defecation in some protozoa, but in other cases they may persist and play a role in aging process. Incomplete digestion may be due to absence of some enzymes, and may lead to accumulation of phospholipids or sphingolipids in some cases and that of glycogen in some other cases. This leads to severe pathologic disturbances.

Autophagic vacuole, also known as cytolysosome or autophagosome, is a lysosome containing a part of the cell itself for digestion. These intracellular parts involved in digestion may include mitochondrion or endoplasmic reticulum and are formed during physiologic and pathologic processes. Under certain conditions, it has been shown that autophagic vacuoles may cause digestion without irreparable damage.

Plant and fungal vacuoles occupying 30-90 per cent of the cell's volume are also comparable to lysosomes of animal cells. They contain hydrolytic enzymes, but perform diverse functions including the following; (i) storage of nutrients and waste products (*e.g.* proteins, anthocyanin, rubber, etc.), (ii) degradation of waste material; (iii) increase of cell size; (iv) control of turgor pressure. The vacuole is also an important homeostatic device so that on drop of pH in the environment, the flux of H^+ into the cytosol, balanced by corresponding transport of H^+ into the vacuole, would keep the pH in the cytosol constant. The turgor pressure of cytosol is similarly maintained by transport of sugars/amino acids, when there is change in osmotic pressure of the fluid surrounding the cell.

Functions: As the word indicates, lysosomes are lytic in nature and are involved in digestion of intracellular or extracellular particles. Depending upon the different kinds of particles described above, following five different functions have been assigned, to lysosomes.

Endocytosis and digestion of macromolecules. The best studied function of lysosomes is the digestion of endocytosed macromolecules. These molecules are initially delivered into early endosomes and then reach late endosomes, before finally reaching the lysosomes.

The hydrolysis starts in the endosomes having a pH of 6.0 and is completed in the lysosomes with a pH of 5.0. A distinction needs to be made between endocytosis and phagocytosis. While endocytosis is a phenomenon common to all cells, phagocytosis is restricted to specialised cells called phagocytes and exemplified by macrophages and neutrophils.

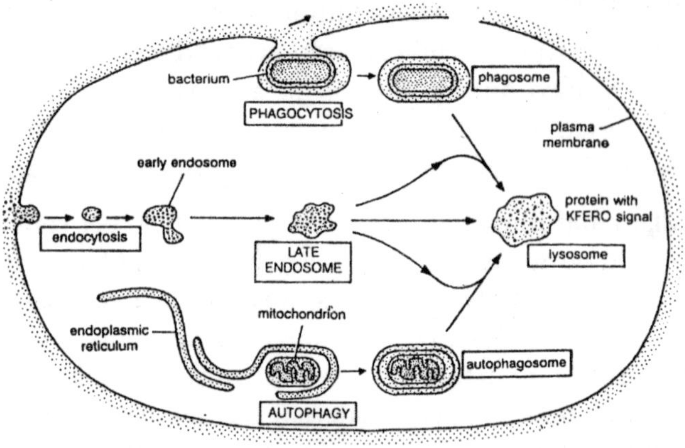

Different stages in the digestion by lysosomes (redrawn from Swanson: The Cell, 1971).

Digestion of External Particles: Large particles and microorganisms are taken into the cell by the process called phagocytosis. The cell engulfs the particles and then forms an invagination that becomes pinched off from the cell membrane and forms an internal sac. Such a sac is known as phagosome. The phagosome moves towards a lysosome and fuses with it to form one structure (Fig.).

The enzymes present in lysosome will then bring about digestion. The lysosome is now called digestive vacuole or secondary lysosome. The residues of digestion are left in the digestive vacuole. The vacuole now moves towards the cell membrane and a process reverse to phagocytosis occurs. Therefore, if the process of digestion has to continue, lysosomes should be produced at the rate of phagocytosis. This process of degradation of large particles, generally occurs in cells specialised for phagocytosis of large particles and microorganisms. Macrophages and neutrophils in vertebrates are the examples of these phagocytes.

Digestion of Intracellular Substances: One of the functions of lysosomes is the digestion of the substances of the same cell to which lysosome belongs. During the process, the substance to be digested penetrates the cell's own lysosomes. The process is known as autophagy (Fig.). For instance, the degeneration of tadpole tail is produced by the action of certain proteolytic enzymes called catepsins contained in lysosomes. There are questions like, what stimulates autophagy? how do the large molecules get into lysosomes?, etc. These questions cannot be easily answered.

Cellular Digestion: When a cell dies, the lysosome membrane ruptures and the enzymes are liberated. These enzymes then digest the dead cell. This is a built-in mechanism of autodigestion to get rid of the cell debris.

Extracellular Digestion: Sometimes a process reverse to phagocytosis occurs and enzymes from a lysosome are liberated outside the cell to which a lysosome and its enzymes belong. It is perhaps through such a mechanism that the sperm penetrates the protective coating of ovum.

For digestion inside the cell, any material to be digested is surrounded by a membrane to form a vacuole or what is described as an endosome. This vacuole or endosome then fuses with a primary or a secondary lysosome where the enzymes bring about digestion. Different kinds of secondary lysosomes fuse and the products of hydrolysis are passed out through the membrane. Resistant material accumulates in the form of residual bodies, which may remain in the cell or discarded out by a process reverse to phagocytosis. Certain food vacuoles have been described in plants which are analogous to lysosomes in function. Lysosomes have been described in certain fungi also.

Origin: In order to absorb a large molecule (a macromolecules the cell wall forms an invagination, which surrounds and encloses the molecule, thus forming an endocytic vesicle (also called endosome) or phagosome. These organelles at this stage do not possess adequate enzymes to digest the enclosed molecule. According to one hypothesis the vesicle travels and comes in contact with Golgi apparatus and derives acid hydrolases from there so that Golgi apparatus should be primarily involved in the formation of lysosomes. According to a modified hypothesis, lysosomes are exclusively formed from Golgi vesicles and the hydrolases synthesized on ribosomes would be subsequently transported through the involvement of endoplasmic reticulum (ER).

Peroxisomes: When improved methods of cell fractionation were available, in addition to lysosomes a second group of particles called peroxisomes were isolated from liver cells. These particles are so called, because they were characterised by their richness in peroxidase, catalase, D-amino acid oxidase and urate oxidase.

Peroxisomes, though commonly found in liver and kidney, are also known from protozoa, yeast and higher plants. In plants following four types of peroxisomes are known: (i) glyoxysomes, (ii) leaf-type peroxisomes, (iii) peroxisomes involved in ureide metabolism, (iv) unspecialised peroxisomes.

Morphology: Peroxisomes, also known as microbodies (discovered by De Duve and his coworkers in 1966), are ovoid granules surrounded by a single membrane. They contain a fine granular substance condensing in centre to form an opaque homogeneous core. The average diameter of a peroxisome in mammalian cells is 0.1 μm to 1.5 μm and their number per cell may range from 70 to 100 as against 15-20 lysosomes per cell. They are particularly abundant in liver and kidney cells.

Peroxisomes differ from mitochondria and chloroplasts in having a single membrane (instead of double membrane) and they do not contain DNA or ribosomes. Since they don't have their own genome, all their proteins must be imported by a process of selective import from cytosol. Thus peroxisomes resemble ER in being self replicating organelles without their own genome.

Import of Proteins into Peroxisomes using a Short Signal Sequence: The contents of peroxisomes are synthesized outside their boundary in the cytosol, because peroxisomes neither have their own genome, nor a protein synthesis machinery. The transport of peroxisomal proteins is facilitated by a specific sequence of three amino acids located near the carboxyl terminus of these proteins. It has been shown that if this sequence of three amino acids is attached to a' cytosolic protein, the protein gets transported to peroxisomes. Importance of this short signal sequence was recognised when its deficiency in patients suffering with the disease Zellweger syndrome, was shown to coexist with the defect in importing proteins into peroxisomes leading to severe protein deficiency in peroxisomes. These patients with empty peroxisomes had severe abnormalities in brain, liver, kidney, so that they died soon after birth.

Functions: Since the peroxisome resembles mitochondrion in utilising oxygen, it has been considered to be a vestige of an ancient organelle, which carried out oxygen metabolism in primitive cells having no mitochondria. It is assumed, according to this hypothesis, that peroxisomes must have served, in the past, the following two functions; (i) lowering of the intracellular concentration of oxygen produced due to photosynthesis, which could have otherwise accumulated to toxic levels; and (ii) carrying out useful oxidative reactions. Later, the development of mitochondria rendered peroxisomes less useful, since their functions were taken over by mitochondria. In mitochondria, these functions are coupled with ATP formation due to oxidative phosphrylation. Peroxisomes, however, still perform some functions-(involving oxidative reactions) not taken over by mitochondria.

Removal of O_2 and Production of H_2O_2: Peroxisomes contain enzymes that use molecular oxygen to remove hydrogen from organic substances and produce hydrogen peroxide. This H_2O_2 is utilised by catalase to oxidise a variety of substances including phenols, formic acid, formaldehyde, and alcohol. Catalase also converts excess H_2O_2 into H_2O.

$$\underset{\substack{\text{organic}\\ \text{Substance}}}{RH_2} + \underset{\substack{\text{molecular}\\ \text{oxygen}}}{O_2} \rightarrow \underset{\substack{\text{hydrogen}\\ \text{peroxide}}}{R + H_2O_2}$$

$$H_2O_2 + R'H_2 \xrightarrow{\text{catalase}} R' + 2H_2O:$$

$$2H_2O_2 \xrightarrow{\text{catalase}} 2H_2O + O_2$$

These oxidative reactions are particularly important in liver and kidney cells for detoxification of various toxic molecules that enter the blood stream. For instance, 25 per cent of ethanol we drink is oxidized to acetaldehyde in this manner.

Breakdown of fatty acids by β oxidation. Breakdown of fatty acid molecules by a process called β oxidation' (in this process alkyl chains of fatty acids are removed sequentially by blocks of two carbon atoms at a time, that are converted to acetyl CoA) is another function of peroxisomes. The acetyl CoA produced during β oxidation is exported from peroxisomes to the cytosol for reuse in biosynthetic pathways. In 'animals this β oxidation occurs both in mitochondira and peroxisomes, while in yeast and plant cells, it occurs only in peroxisomes.

Photorespiration and glyoxylate cycle. In plants two types of peroxisomes perform following two different but important functions: (i) In leaves, leaf-type peroxisomes help in photorespiration (involving oxidation of a side product of photosynthesis) in which O_2 is used and CO_2 is liberated; (ii) In germinating seeds, they convert fatty acids into sugars (needed for the growth of the young plant) by a series of reactions known as glyoxylate cycle, so that these peroxisomes are called glyoxysomes. In this glyoxylate cycle, two molecules of acetyl CoA produced due to breakdown of fatty acid β oxidation) are used to make succinic acid which leaves peroxisomes and gets converted into glucose. This glyoxylate cycle does not occur in animals, so that they are incapable of converting fatty acids (found in fats) into sugars.

Enzymes and Diseases Caused by their Deficiency: Peroxisome membrane contains two major (22K, 70K; K= kilo daltons) and several less abundant peroxisome specific proteins. The organelle matrix has more than 40 enzymes, which catalyze a variety of reactions.

These reactions can be anabolic (*e.g.* plasminogen biosynthesis, bile acid biosynthesis) or catabolic (P oxidation of very long chain fatty acids or VLCFA; H_2O_2 based respiration). The H_2O_2 metabolism utilises three enzymes (urate oxidase, D-amino oxidase and α-hydroxylic acid oxidase) in production of H_2O_2 and a fourth enzyme (catalase) in its degradation. There are also interactions between intra-peroxisomal reactions and extra-peroxisomal pathways, needing transport of metabolites across peroxisome membrane (Fig.).

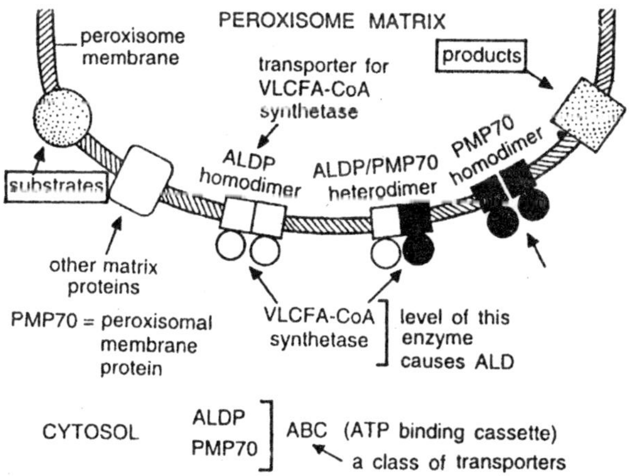

The role of different peroxisome membrane proteins, particularly in H_2O_2 metabolism, intra-peroxisomal reactions and in extra-peroxisomal pathways.

Peroxisomes' are also responsible for certain diseases (as shown in early 1990s). These diseases can be broadly classified into two types: (i) diseases due to deficiency of a specific matrix enzyme (single enzyme deficiency), like ALD (adrenoleukodystrophy) and (ii) diseases due to defects in the formation of the organelle (inborn errors of peroxisome biogenesis), like Zellweger syndrome.

In ALD disease (which is most common inherited peroxisomal disease), at mid-childhood, there is onset of insufficiency of VLCFA-CoA synthetase (VLCFA = very long chain fatty acids). It has been shown that ALD is caused due to defect in a protein' ALDP (having homology to a 70K peroxisomal protein PMP70, rather than to the expected VLCFA-CoA synthetase), which is involved in the transport of VLCFA-CoA synthetase across the peroxisome membrane. ALDP belongs to ATP binding cassette (ABC) transporter protein super-family.

Origin: Earlier, it was believed that the peroxisomes originate by budding from the ER and that its contents were imported from the cytosol. However, evidence is now available to suggest that new peroxisomes arise only from pre-existing peroxisomes by growth and fusion.

Hydrogenosome: Another, eukaryotic organelle, the hydrogenosome was identified in the year 1997. It is endosymbiotic in its origin, and is entirely dependent on the nucleus for its genetic livelihood; during late 1998, a genome was also shown to be present in the hydrogenosome of a ciliate *Nycototherus ovalis.* Although, hydrogenosome occur widely, its history is elucidated only in trichomonads (parasitic flagellated protists).

These anaerobes (which can though live in air) lack mitochondria and peroxisomes, and instead possess hydrogenosomes, the unusual energy generating organelles. In *Trichomonas,* the hydrogenosome has been shown to be a derived mitochondrion. Like mitochondria, hydrogenosomes have each a double membrane envelope, divide autonomously by fission, import protein post-translationally and produce ATP by substrate-level phosphorylation. They differ from mitochondria in lacking (i) cytochromes, (ii) tricarboxylic acid (TCA) cycle and (iii) oxidative phosphorylation.

They use enzymes typical of anaerobes (*e.g.* pyruvate : ferredoxin oxidoreductase and hydrogenase), and they produce large quantities of hydrogen giving them the name hydrogenosome.

Two hypotheses have been proposed for the origin of trichomonad hydrogenosome. It may either be the product of an independent endosymbiosis of an anaerobic eubacterium or it may be a highly modified mitochondrion adapted to an anaerobic lifestyle.

The latter hypothesis is now strongly supported by the demonstration that the *Trichomonas* nucleus carries genes for one or all the three of the mitochondrial heat-shock proteins (Hsp 10, Hsp 60, Hsp 70) although only Hsp 60 and Hsp 70 reside in hydrogenosome. These Hsp proteins are considered to be the most reliable traces of the eubacterial origin in both, the mitochondrion and the chloroplast.

Hydrogenosomes are found in a variety of unrelated anaerobic or microaerobic eukaryotes, which are all devoid of mitochondria. These include a variety of ciliates, certain rumen fungi and some percolozoan protists. The hydrogenosomes of these organisms are derived either from mitochondria or from peroxisomes. Recent studies also suggest that mitochondrion was present in the ancestors of all extant eukaryotes and that subsequent evolution was reductive, not acquistive (with the exception of chloroplasts) so that the hydrogenosome was derived from the mitochondrion (or peroxisome) due to loss of genome as a consequence of the loss of respiration. However, in the chloroplast, loss of photosynthesis does not lead to loss of genome, because it performs functions other than photosynthesis as well (Fig.).

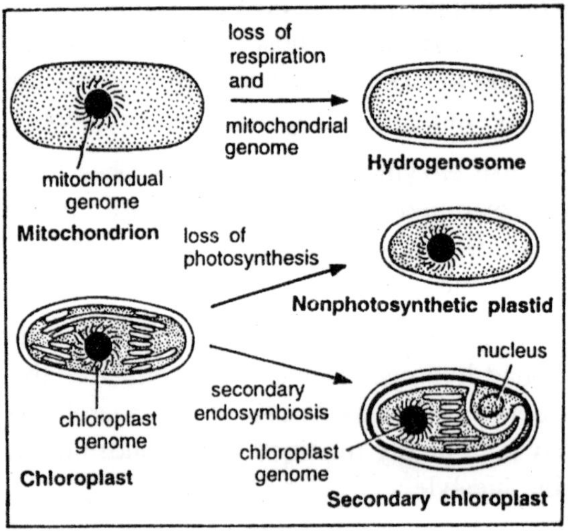

Origin of hydrogenosome from mitochondria and those of non-photosynthetic plastids and secondary chloroplasts from photosynthetic chloroplasts (redrawn from Science, 7 February. 1997).

Centrosome: The term 'centrosome' *(centrosome* = central body) was coined by T. Boveri in 1888 for an organelle that occupies a central position in interphase cells. It is from this organelle that the spindle fibres radiate as an aster in mitosis in the cells of animals and lower plants. Despite its significance in the division of animal cells, it is generally absent in cells of higher plants.

Structure: Each centrosome contains two centrioles (diplosomes), surrounded by an amorphous cloud of pericentriolar material (PCM) also described as centrosphere. Within the PCM is located a Kl-insoluble structure called 'centromatrix,' which functions as a scaffold for the binding of 25-nm ring shaped protein complexes, called γ -tubulin ring complexes (γ -TuRCs), made up of γ -tubulin and several other proteins including pericentrin, centrin, centrosomin and ninein. Centrosome's ability to nucleate microtubules, which is described as microtubule nucleation potential (MNP), resides in these protein complexes.

Each centriole looks like a cylinder which is about 300-500 nm in length and 150-180 nm in diameter. The wall of each cylinder or centriole contains 9 triplet fibres, arranged around a central axis. Each triplet fibre consists of three secondary fibres or tubules 20 nm in diameter. The three tubules are arranged in a line tilted at about 40° to the tangent of the centriole. (Fig.).

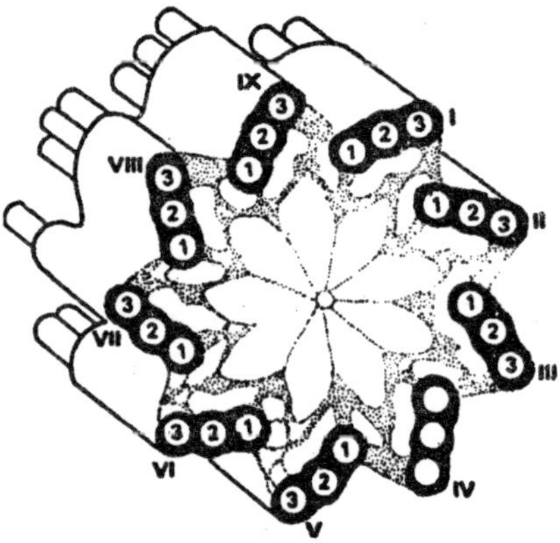

Three dimensional view of a centriole (in front is the sectional view).

There is evidence for the presence of DNA and RNA in centrioles. Probably the information for the synthesis of centrioles is derived from a tiny DNA containing unit with about 2×10^{-16} g double stranded DNA.

Function: The centrosome is implicated in the formation of the basal bodies, spindle fibres, cilia, etc. As the time of cell division approaches, the centrioles separate and move to opposite poles of the nucleus. Spindle is formed between them and the chromosomes become arranged at the equator. With the help of the spindle fibres attached to the centromeres of the chromosomes, the latter are dragged towards the poles, perhaps due to the contraction of the spindle fibre.

Centrosome and Cancer: Recently, two human serine/ threonine kinases (STK15, aurora2), that are found associated with the centrosome have been shown to be amplified in human cancers, which carried cells with increased number of centrosomes and aneuploidy. Similar proteins associated with centrosome dysfunction are also known in fruitfly and yeast. It is hypothesized, that increased kinase activity results in centrosome defects, which lead to aberrant mitotic spindles, mis-segregation of chromosomes and aneuploidy thus causing cancerous growth of cells.

Origin: The origin of centrosome is mainly through the replication of centrioles which are semi-autonomous. Replication of centrioles, whereby each centriole gives rise to an additional daughter centriole begins when the centrioles separate. The daughter centrioles arise as 'procentrioles' from the side of a pre-existing centriole close to one end and grow to mature size in late prophase maintaining their close proximity to and orientation at right angles to the mother centriole. Consequently when the interphase nuclei reform at the end of a nuclear division, a centrosome containing two centrioles is again found besides each nucleus.

6

Cell Division

Development of an organism from the zygote to the full grown stage takes place by the division of cells. Even after full size has been attained, replacement of cells takes place by cell division. The process of *cell division whereby the chromosomes are duplicated and distributed equally to the daughter cells is called mitosis*.

The mitotic cycle is divided into many phases: *prophase, prometaphase, metaphase, anaphase* and *telophase*. The period between two mitotic cycles is called *interphase*.

Interphase: This is the so called 'resting stage,' but is in fact a period of great activity. Three important processes which are preparatory to cell division take place during interphase: (1) *Replication of DNA* takes place, and also the *synthesis* of basic nuclear proteins, the histones. (2) The *centrioles divide*, forming a pair of new centrioles, which are at right angles to each other. Reproduction of a centriole takes place by the outgrowth of daughter centrioles from the parent centrioles. (3) *Synthesis of energy-rich compounds* which provide energy for mitosis, and *synthesis of proteins* which are later found in the spindle, takes place at the end of interphase.

Interphase can be divided into three periods (Fig.B). (1) The *post-mitotic gap phase* (G1) takes place at the end of one cell division. RNA and proteins are synthesized during this period, but there is no synthesis of DNA. (2) During the *synthesis phase* (S) DNA is formed from purine and pyrimidine nucleotides. During this period the DNA content of the nucleus is doubled. (3) During the *pre-mitotic gap phase* (G2), synthesis of RNA and protein continues, but DNA synthesis stops. The time taken for the S phase, the G2 phase and mitosis is approximately equal. The length of G1 is usually greater, and is also subjected to greater variation. Cells which do not divide frequently have a longer G1 phase, while frequently dividing cells have a shorter phase. The G1 phase can be terminated by various stimuli, and cell division then starts. Once a cell has entered the S phase and has begun DNA replication, it has usually committed itself to division.

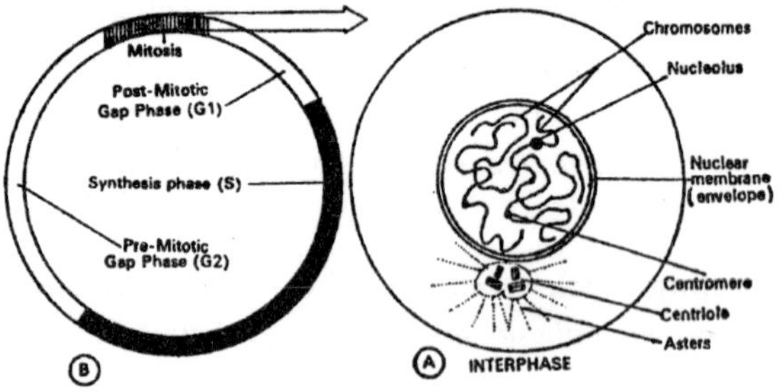

(A) The cell during interphase (B) The cell cycle.

During interphase, duplication of the chromosomes takes place. Each chromosome (called the *monad)* becomes double, and is then called the *dyad*.

Prophase: During prophase, the cell becomes spheroid, and there is increase in viscosity and refractivity. The chromosomes shorten and thicken and become stainable. By the end of prophase, some chromosomes may contract to 1/25 of their length in early prophase. The double nature of the chromosomes is now visible. Each chromosome consists of two *chromatids* united by a *centromere,* and is called a dyad. With the progress of prophase, the chromosomes which were evenly distributed in early prophase migrate towards the nuclear membrane, leaving a clear central area.

The centrioles, which had undergone duplication during interphase, now begin to move towards opposite poles of the cell. This movement is due to their being pushed apart by growth of the spindle fibres between them. Taylor has shown that in newts, the centrioles move at a velocity of one micron per minute. In animal cells and cells of lower plants, fibrils appear like spokes of a wheel around each centriole to form an *aster.* The asters are cytoplasmic in origin.

When the centriole is present and participates in cell division, mitosis is said to be *centric.* In species which do not have centrioles mitosis is said to be *acentric.* Cell division in which the aster is formed is called *astral mitosis* e. g. animals and lower plants. Centrioles may be present without the aster, in which case mitosis is said to be *anastral, e.g.* higher plants. Centric mitosis may be astral or anastral.

The spindle begins to be formed between the two poles. It is formed mainly from nuclear material. It is gel-like in nature with a limited rigidity. The spindle consists of *microtubules* about 250A in diameter. The microtubules are cylinders formed from protein monomers. The number of microtubules varies from 16 in yeast cells to 5000 in higher plants.

The aster, the centrioles and the spindle together make up the mitotic apparatus or *achromatic figure.*

Two types of spindles have been described, the *central* spindle and the *metaphasic* spindle. During the formation of the *central* spindle, the centrosome divides into two at the beginning of prophase. Each body gives off astral rays to form *asters, and the* spindle is formed between them. In the *metaphasic* spindle, the centrioles divide and form asters before the beginning of prophase. Spindle formation, however, takes place when the chromosomes begin their metaphasic movements.

Prometaphase: The beginning of prometaphase is marked by the disappearance of the nuclear membrane. When the nuclear membrane dissolves, there is no differentiation between cytoplasm and nucleoplasm. Such mitosis is called *extranuclear* mitosis or *eumitosis*. In many Protozoa and some animal cells, however, the nuclear membrane does not disappear during cell division. Mitosis takes place within the nuclear membrane and is called *intranuclear* mitosis or *premitosis*. In some protists, the centriole is within the nucleus. In such cases mitosis is both *intranuclear* and *centric*. When the centriole is outside the nucleus mitosis is *extranuclear* and *centric*.

When the nuclear membrane dissolves, a fluid area is observed in the centre of the cell. The chromosomes move freely through this area as they proceed towards the equator.

Metaphase: At metaphase the chromosomes have reached the central or equatorial portion of the spindle. They are lined up in one place to form the *equatorial plate* or *metaphasic plate*. The centrioles lie on the equator of the spindle. Usually the arms of the chromosomes lie on the equator of spindle. Occasionally, only the centromeres lie on the equatorial plane and the arms are directed towards the poles. Chromosomes are irregularly arranged on the equatorial plane in plant cells. Smaller chromosomes are usually central in position while larger ones are peripheral.

There is evidence that the spindle fibres are definite structures. Taylor reports that when a microdissection needle is inserted into the cell it can be moved freely along the longitudinal axis, but meets resistance when moved transversely. This indicates that longitudinal fibrils are present. There are two types of spindle fibres. *Continuous* fibres extend from pole to pole (Fig. A). They form the *stemkorper* or pushing body in animal cells. Later on *interzonal* fibres are found between the chromosomes. *Chromosomal* fibres extend from the pole to the centromere of the chromosome. Spindles are of two types, *direct* and *indirect*. In the *direct* type, chromosomal fibres connect the chromosomes directly with the pole (Fig. B). In the *indirect* (Fig. C) type the chromosomes are connected with the continuous fibres.

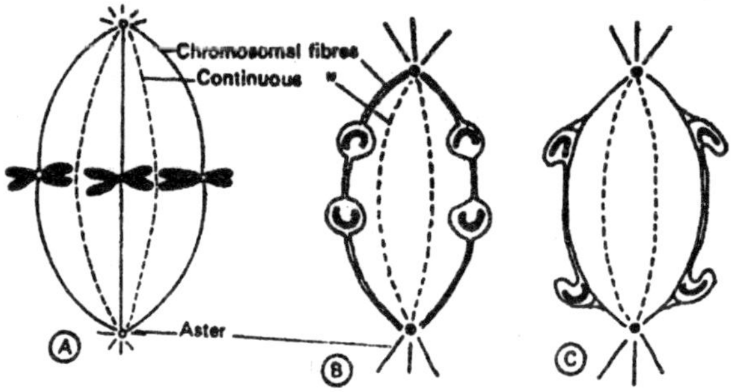

(A) Metaphasic spindle. (B) Direct spindle. (C) Indirect spindle.

RNA synthesis ceases during metaphase and anaphase.

Anaphase: The chromosomes are arranged on the equatorial plate for a short period only. The centromeres of the chromosomes divide simultaneously as anaphase commences, and the two chromatids of each pair separate. They are now called *daughter chromosomes*.

The daughter chromosomes now behave as if they repel each other. The two sets of chromosomes migrate towards the poles. The forces behind chromosome movement are not yet known.

Various theories have been suggested for the migration of chromosomes, *e.g.* pulling by contraction of spindle fibres, pushing by expansion of the fibres, a combination of contraction and expansion, viscosity changes in the cell, electrostatic forces, diffusion currents, viscous streaming of protoplasm, hydrodynamic forces and tactoids.

The most widely held view is that the spindle fibres attached to the centromeres shorten and pull the chromosomes to the poles. Simultaneously the fibres between the two poles lengthen and push the poles apart.

Do the spindle fibres attached to the centromeres of the chromosomes contract and pull the chromosomes to the poles? A fact cited in favour of this view is that the chromosomes become V-shaped with their arms trailing as they travel towards the poles. Another point is that centromeres are essential for chromosome movement. Chromosomes which have lost their centromeres, or parts of chromosomes without centromeres, fail to move to the poles.

However, there is also evidence to the contrary. If chromosomal fibres contract, they should become thicker and shorter. They have not been observed to become thicker. Secondly, it has been found in experiments with amoebae that when spindle fibres are cut with microneedles, the chromosomes still migrate normally.

In certain cells, the aster rays are attached to the cell membrane. It was believed that the rays anchor the poles to the membrane during chromosome movement. It has, however, been shown experimentally that the chromosomes move to the poles even when the aster rays are broken by a microneedle. Therefore, the view that the rays anchor the poles is no longer valid.

In spite of the objections mentioned above it is believed that the chromosomes are pulled by spindle fibres. It is explained that the fibres do not become thicker when they shorten because they dissolve progressively in the region of the centriole. Chromosomal movement according to this view is thus due to shortening (not contraction) of spindle fibres. Shortening of the chromosomal fibres is by slow removal of protein monomers from the polar region. Elongation of continuous fibres results from addition of new monomers.

The velocity of chromosomal movement ranges from 0.2 μ m per minute to about 5 μ m per minute. The rate of movement is independent of the size of the chromosomes. Sister chromatids move to opposite poles with similar velocities, but these need not be identical. All the chromosomes of a cell move towards the poles simultaneously, except for the sex chromosomes, which frequently lag behind. Sometimes a particular chromosome may move in advance. The chromosomes move at a deaccelerating rate, never at an accelerating rate.

Telophase: Telophase changes are associated with the restoration of the interphase condition. In a way telophase is the reverse of prophase. Telophase begins when the two sets of daughter chromosomes reach opposite poles of the cell. The gel of the spindle reverts to the sol state and the spindle disappears.

A new *nuclear membrane* is formed around each set of chromosomes. The nucleoli reappear at constrictions, called the *nucleolar organisers,* in one pair of chromosomes. Each daughter cell gets the same complement of nucleoli at the same sites as did the parent cell. The chromosomes gradually uncoil and become less compact. They eventually lose their ability to stain.

Cytokinesis: In animal cells a *cleavage furrow* appears at the beginning of telophase. This furrow or constriction becomes progressively deeper as the spindle breaks down. Eventually the ingrowing constrictions join and separate two daughter cells. This division is called *cytokinesis.* If nuclear division takes place without cytoplasmic division, a *syncytium* is formed. In plants there is a formation of a *cell plate* between the two groups of chromosomes. The cell plate grows from the middle towards the periphery, and finally joins the cell wall. The early cell plate is the middle lamella of the many layered cell wall.

During division, cell organelles like mitochondria, plastids, Golgi complex, lysosomes and the cytoplasmic matrix are distributed to the two daughter cells. Of these, mitochondria and plastids reproduce themselves, but details of the other organelles are not known.

Importance of Somatic Cell Division

Equal Distribution of Chromosomes: The essential feature of mitosis is that chromosomes are distributed equally among the two daughter cells. With every cell division there is a division of chromosomes. Repeated division, by mitosis from the zygote onwards ensures an identical genetic constitution for all the cells of the body. The constant number of chromosomes in all the cells of the body is because of mitosis.

Surface-volume Ratio: Mitosis restores the surface-volume ratio of the cell. A small cell has a greater amount of surface available in relation to volume that a large cell. As the cell increases in size, the available surface area in relation to increased volume becomes less. By undergoing division, the cell becomes smaller in size and the surface-volume ratio is restored.

Nucleoplasmic Index: The growth of a multicellular organism is due to mitosis. A cell cannot grow in size to a large extent without disturbing the ratio between the nucleus and the cytoplasm. After a particular size has been reached, the cell divides to restore the *nucleo plasmic index.* Thus growth takes place by an increase in the number of cells, rather than by increase in the size of the cells. An idea of growth due to mitosis can be obtained from the fact that the human body contains 60,000,000,000,000, cells, all ultimately derived by division of a single cell. Repair of the body takes place because of addition of cells by mitosis. Dead cells of the upper layer of the epidermis, cells of the lining of the gut, and red blood corpuscles are constantly being replaced. It is estimated that in the human body about 500,000,000,000, cells are lost daily.

Breakdown of the Nuclear Envelope: The nucleus is bounded by a double nuclear envelope in which are several nuclear pore complexes. During prophase the nuclear envelope may break down into several pieces, or may form small vesicles. In *Chaetopterus*, the breakdown takes about two minutes. Pieces of the nuclear envelope or the pore complexes may disappear, or may persist throughout mitosis. During telophase, the pieces are used in the reformation of the nuclear envelope. It has been suggested that a histone fraction released by DNA weakens the nuclear envelope before it is broken down. The actual breakdown of the envelope, however, is apparently due to it being pulled and pushed by the microtubules of the spindle fibres.

The Spindle

The existence of the spindle was for long debated and it was considered by some to be a fixation artifact. However, its presence has now been confirmed. The evidence is based on the facts (1) that the spindle is visible under the phase contrast and polarising microscopes, (2) that it can be displaced by ultracentrifugation, and (3) that it has been possible to isolate it from many cells. The presence of the spindle is essential for mitosis. If cells are treated with *colchicine*, which inhibits spindle formation, anaphasic movement of the two groups of chromosomes to the poles does not take place. The spindle is largely a protein gel. ATPase activity has been associated with the spindle, suggesting a contractile mechanism similar to that of muscle fibres, although the load on the spindle is much less. There is no evidence that the spindle is bounded by a membrane. The spindle is a dynamic structure, and undergoes a cycle of dissolution and re-formation.

Types of Spindles: There are two types of spindles, *anastral* and *astral*. The *anastral* spindle is without centrioles, blepharoplasts or asters. It is typically found in higher plants, but has also been reported in several animal ova and Protista. Usually the spindle is *symmetrical*, and consists of two equal half-spindles. In some cases, however, *e.g.* in dividing pollen, the spindle poles are *non-symmetrical,* one pole is diffuse and the other pointed. One group of chromsomes may therefore converge towards the spindle pole, while the other group diverges. In the *anastral* spindle, the spindle fibres radiate from spindle poles or centrioles.

Spindle Fibres: Three types of spindle fibres have been distinguished, *chromosomal fibres, continuous fibres* and *interzonal fibres. Chromosomal fibres* extend from the *kinetochore (centromere)* to the pole of the spindle. They shorten during cell division and pull the daughter chromosomes apart. They are formed by the centromeres of the chromosomes. The microtubules, of which the fibres are composed, grow continuously from the kinetochores to the poles during prometaphase and metaphase. Continuous fibres extend from pole to pole without attaching to the chromosomes. They elongate during cell division and push the spindle poles apart, thus separating the chromosomes. The fibres form between the poles, regardless of whether chromosomes are present or not. They are formed even after the chromosomes are removed by microsurgery.

Microtubules: Electron microscope studies show that the spindle fibre consists of a bundle of *microtubules* embedded in a protein matrix. Microtubules are long cylinders, about 250A in diameter. A section through the cylinder shows that it is hollow. The wall of the cylinder is electron-dense and is approximately 50-70A thick. The wall appears to be made up of 13 longitudinally arranged *filamentous subunits* with a centre-to-centre spacing of 50A. The filaments appear to be made up of small *monomers* of globular protein (*tubulin)* about 40-50A in diameter. It is believed that *monomers* form *dimers* through disulphide linkages. The dimers polymerise to form *filaments,* which then aggregate to form *microtubules.*

Regularly spaced *side arms* or *cross bridges* have been observed between the microtubules of the spindle. McIntosh (1968) has speculated that the side arms may be arranged in a regular manner, every 30° around the microtubules, forming a helix. The side arms at once bring to mind the connections between microtubules in cilia and flagella, and the cross bridges between myosin and actin filaments in muscle fibres. This has led to the suggestion that a uniform contraction model for both muscle and spindle is possible.

It appears that the spindle is organised from a pre-existing pool of protein. It is postulated that protein monomers aggregate to form microtubules of the spindle fibres. The spindle fibres are thus oriented polymers. It has been proposed that the continuous fibres are *elongated* by the insertion of subunits within the fibre. This leads to the elongation of the spindle. Conversely, the *shortening* of chromosomal fibres takes place by loss of subunits. This de-polymerisation of fibres takes place in the region of the spindle poles. Thus the fibres do not *contract* like a rubber band, but *shorten* by loss of material at one end. This is in agreement with observations that no change in the thickness of fibres takes place during shortening and elongation. There is evidence that the microtubules of the chromosomal fibres originate at the kinetochore. Microtubules are also found in cells which have no centrioles, e. g. those of higher plants. Here the microtubules end in the pole region and are not attached anywhere.

Kinetochore (Centromere)

Under the electron microscope, the kinetochore of most higher plants appears as a diffuse ball with a denser core. Microtubules of spindle fibres can be seen attached to the kinetochore. In higher animals the structure of the kinetochore is different. The kinetochore of prometaphase and telophase appears to be composed of three zones:

(1) an *outer dense zone* composed of a pair of coiled axial fibrils 50-80A in diameter, according to one interpretation,

(2) an *inner zone* next to the chromosome body, and

(3) a lighter *intermediate zone* consisting of loops from the axial fibres.

Microtubules have been found embedded in all the three layers or in the outer layer. A similar structure has been found in some lower plants (e. g. the alga *Oedogonium).* On the other hand, lower animals like cockroaches and sea urchins do not show the three zones. According to another interpretation (Luykx, 1970), the kinetochore is composed of a series of *discs.* These discs are attached to the primary constriction. Several microtubules are attached to each kinetochore. In many insects and in some algae the kinetochores are *diffused.* In such cases the microtubules connect throughout the length of the chromosome. During anaphase, such chromosomes are not bent at an angle but move in a parallel manner.

Kinetochores have not been observed during interphase, and probably develop in the early stages of chromosome differentiation. According to one suggestion, the kinetochores are products of genes, and their activity is genetically controlled. The kinetochores have two functions. The main function apparently is that they serve for the *attachment of microtubules* of the chromosomal spindle fibres. They might also be involved in the *formation of the chromosomal spindle fibres* during prometaphase and metaphase by serving as centres for polymerisation of the protein of microtubules.

Anaphasic Motion

Several hypotheses have been put forward to explain the movement of chromosomes during anaphase. These include the pulling of chromosomes by contraction of spindle fibres, pushing by expansion of fibres, a combination of contraction and expansion, viscosity changes in the cell, electrostatic forces, diffusion currents, viscous streaming of protoplasm, hydrodynamic forces and tactoids. A brief review will be made of the various hypotheses before current views are dealt with. Electrostatic force. Lillie (1905) advanced the idea that chromosomal movement is the result of an electrical charge. The cytoplasm was considered to be electronegative, and the nuclear contents, with the exception of the chromosomes, electropositive. The chromosomes were considered to be electronegative. Although the cell does have different areas with different electrical charges, this theory cannot account for many of the exceptional cases of mitosis, and also becomes very complicated when applied to meiosis.

Hydrodynamics: This theory was put forward by the physicist Bjerknes (1902, 1909). The essential features of the theory are as follows: (1) Two pulsating spheres in a liquid medium attract each other when they pulsate in phase, and repulse each other when they pulsate in opposite phase, (2) Such pulsating spheres set up hydrodynamic lines of force resembling electrical or magnetic fields. (3) A neutral sphere in such a field is repelled if it is lighter than the medium and attracted if it is heavier. (4) In the cell, the spindle poles are supposed to represent the pulsating spheres and the chromosomes the heutral sphere. Changes in the specific gravity of the chromosomes determine whether the chromosomes will be attracted or repelled. This theory does not account for the formation of the metaphasic plate. It also seems unlikely that the forces can operate at the distances where the chromosomes and spindle poles are situated.

Tactoids: When long fibres are suspended in an unoriented medium, they show a tendency to line up in a spindle form. Several workers, e. g. Bernal (1940), Ostergren (1945) and Schrader (1951) have attempted to explain anaphasic movement on the basis of this fact. However, there is insufficient physiochemical data for the acceptance of the role of tactoids in mitosis.

Streaming Currents: According to the theory proposed by

Schaede (1929-30), chromosomes are repelled to the equatorial plate during prometaphase by viscous streams from the poles. During anaphase a reverse streaming towards the poles results in anaphasic movements of chromosomes. The spindle fibres were thought to be lamellar streams of viscous protoplasm. The fact that the spindle fibres consist of definite microtubules makes this theory untenable.

Current Views: Electron microscope studies have shown that the spindle fibres are composed of microtubules. These in turn are composed of 13 filaments arranged in a ring. Each filament consists of linearly arranged protein monomers. Chromosome movements take place by the action of either the chromosomal spindle fibres, or the continuous spindle fibres, or by the action of both: (1) In some Orthopteran insects, chromosome movements takes place by simultaneous shortening of chromosomal fibres and elongation of continuous fibres. (2) In some Homoptera, even though both movements are present they occur separately. (3) In one aphid species, chromosome movement appears to take place by elongation of the continuous fibres *only*, even though chromosomal fibres are also present. (4) In some plant cells with rigid cell walls, spindle enlargement is not possible. Chromosomal movement takes place entirely by shortening of chromosomal fibres. (5) In most organisms there is an initial shortening of chromosomal fibres, followed by elongation of the spindle.

As mentioned previously, elongation of continuous fibres takes place by insertion of subunits within the fibre. Shortening conversely takes place by loss of subunits in the region of the spindle poles. These processes recall the old contraction and expansion theories (Klein, 1878-79; Van Beneden, 1883) but there is a basic difference. If chromosomes were to be pulled by *contraction* of spindle fibres, in the way a rubber band contracts, then one would expect the fibres to become thicker. However, it has been observed that there is no change in the thickness of the fibres during shortening and elongation. This would be quite in agreement with the view that shortening of fibres takes place by loss of material at the poles.

Process of Division

There are two types of cell divisions, somatic cell division or mitosis and the reduction division or meiosis. Mitotic cell division involves a single cell division cycle producing two daughter cells genetically identical not only to each other, but also to the parent cell. Meiotic cell division, on the other hand, involves pairing of homologous chromosomes and recombination associated with two cell division cycles producing four daughter cells, genetically different not only among themselves, but also from the parent cell.

The success of mitotic cell division depends on faithful alternation of chromosome replication (S phase) and chromosome segregation (M phase). Similarly, the success of meiotic cell division depends on faithful chromosome replication and pairing of homologous chromosomes, followed by the segregation of these chromosomes at the two successive cell division cycles. The events that control the above events during mitosis and meiosis are genetically controlled and have been studied at the molecular level, so that one could ask questions such as the following: what are the factors which order a particular cell to undergo cell division, mitosis or meiosis? Does the mechanism of cell division involve a mere difference between interphase and mitosis/meiosis or is it much more complicated? Are there specific genes and gene products which, regulate and control orderly sequence of events in a cell division cycle? Significant progress has been made in recent years (1980's and 1990's) to answer these questions.

A study of the mechanism of cell division is also important for finding solutions to uncontrolled cell division in cancerous tissues. In recognition of the significance of the study of regulation of cell division cycle in treatment of cancer, the Nobel Prize in Medicine or Physiology for the year 2001 was awarded to Paul Nurse and Thomas Hunt of UK and Leland Hartmann of USA. While P. Nurse and L. Hartmann discovered genes *(cdc, CDC)* for cyclin dependent kinases (Cdks) in two yeasts, T. Hunt discovered cyclins in sea urichin, yeasts and mammals. These different aspects involving a study of genetics and biochemistry of cell division will be discussed in this chapter.

Genetic Vs. Biochemical Approaches for the Study of Cell Division Cycle: Following two approaches have been used for the study of the control of cell division cycle: (i) Geneticists analysed mutations that arrested the cell division cycle of somatic cells (excluding embryonic cells) at specific points (particularly in yeast).

Most cell cycle mutatnts would be generally lethal. Therefore, for the study of cell cycle, conditional mutants were isolated, which will express under one condition and can be maintained in the other alternative condition. Temperature sensitive mutants is an example of such conditional mutants.

They express the mutant state at one temperature (*e.g.*, 36°C) and continue normal cell division at another temperature (*e.g.*, 23°C). This approach allowed the identification of genes involved in the cell-cycle control system, (ii) Physiologists, biochemists and embryologists, on the other hand, analysed the points of arrest of the cell cycle and used agents that restored the normal cell cycle.

For this approach, embryonic cell divisions in sea urchin and frog *(Xenopus)* eggs were often used, since embryonic cells undergo rapid cell divisions and are, therefore, the simplest systems for a study of cell cycle. In this approach, cell cycle is described as a biochemical machine (having two states) that oscillates between interphase and mitosis. This approach allowed identification of chemical compounds (including enzymes) that regulate and control the cell division cycle. Initially these two approaches and theories seemed incompatible, but recently these could be used to present a unified picture to explain the mechanism of cell division.

Yeast and Somatic Cell Division

Genetic investigations on cell division have been conducted on yeasts, *Drosophila* and *Aspergillus*, but the most important of these studies were conducted on two yeasts, the budding yeast *(Saccharomyces cerevisiae)* and the fission yeast *(Schizosaccharomyces pombe)*.

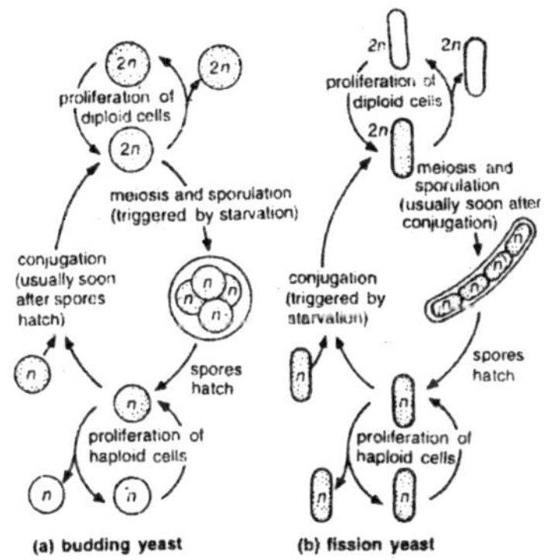

The life cycles of a budding yeast (Saccharomyces cerevisiae) and fission yeast (Schizosaccharomyces pombe); note that under supply of plentiful nutrients, budding yeast proliferates as diploid cells, while fission years proliferates as haploid cells; some widely used strains of budding yeast also proliferate as haploid cells (redrawn from Alberts et. al., Molecular Biology of the Cell', 1994).

The life cycles of these two yeasts are though largely similar (Fig.), there are also differences. For instance, in fission yeast the elongated cells divide by fission, but in budding yeast, cells divide by forming a bud. There seems to be no G2 phase in budding yeast (Fig.). In both these yeasts, a large collection of cell division cycle mutants (genes are designated as *cdc* in fission yeast; *CDC* in budding yeast) were isolated, which arrest the cell cycle at specific points described as checkpoints.

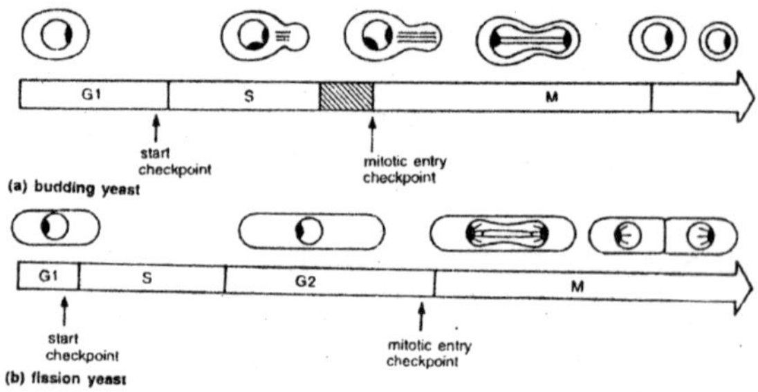

A comparison of the cell cycles of fission yeast and budding yeast; note the absence of G2 phase in budding yeast; unlike higher eukaryotes, the nuclear envelope does not break in either case (redrawn from Alberts et. al., 'Molecular Biology of the Cell', 1994).

The interactions of these mutants were analysed and the products of mutant genes were compared with the macro-molecules isolated and studied by those who studied the biochemistry of the cell division. About 80 *cdc/CDC* genes have been identified in each of these two species, although all of them are not involved in regulation of the cell division cycle. Some of these genes are listed in Table.

Some Yeast Cell-division-cycle Genes and their Functions

Gene name in budding yeast	*Gene name in fission yeast*	*Gene product*	*Phenotype of loss-of function mutant*
CDC2	*po13*	Catalytic subunit of DNA polymerase 8	Arrest in S phase
CDC9	*cdc17*	DNA ligase	Arrest in G_2 with imperfectly replicated DNA
CDC28	*cdc2*	Serine/threonine protein kinase	Arrest at 'start' or at mitotic entry (G_2) checkpoint
SWI6	*cdc10*	Gene regulatory protein required for transcription of G_1 cyclins	Failure to enter S phase

Contd....

Gene name in budding yeast	*Gene name in fission yeast*	*Gene product*	*Phenotype of loss-of function mutant*
CLN 1,2,3	?	G_1 cyclins	Arrest at 'start' (if all three genes inactive)
CLB 1,2,3,4	*cdc* 13	Mitotic cyclins	Arrest at mitotic entry (G_2) checkpoint
WEE1	*weel*	Tyrosine protein kinase	Premature passage past mitotic entry (G_2) checkpoint, hence small size
MIH1	*cdc25*	Tyrosine protein phosphatase	Arrest at mitotic entry (G_2) checkpoint
RAD9	?	Protein of unknown function (loss of feedback control)	Failure to delay mitosis when DNA is damaged
D1S2, SI	*dis2*	Protein phosphatase I	Arrest in mitosis

The Gl phase of the mitotic cell division cycle in yeast has been divided into pre-start Gl, start and post-start Gl stages.

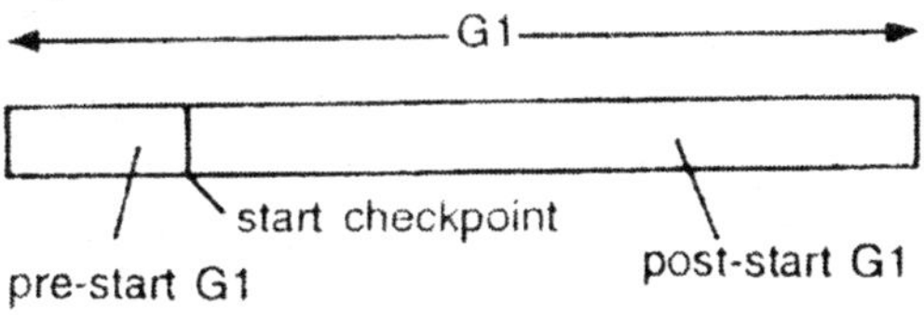

Gl phase of the cell cycle in yeasts, showing pre-start Gl, start and post-start Gl phases.

In the cell cycle of budding yeast, 'start' is particularly an important control point, where the mating pheromones (α factor and *a* factor produced by the α and *a* mating types respectively) cause cell cycle arrest, allowing cells to undergo conjugation. In mammals, passage of the cell cycle through 'start' (also called restriction point) requires that:

(i) the cell attains a minimum size, so that unless this size is attained, the cell cycle will not proceed beyond 'pre-start Gl';

(ii) the cells are not in short supply of nutrients, so that if the cells are starved, they will not pass through 'start', even after attaining the required minimum size;

(iii) the cells do not have any mating 'pheromones' and are thus not made to, undergo conjugation. Mutants have been isolated, which mimic defects in all these different conditions.

Differentiation in Somatic Cell Cycle

There are also variations in the cell division cycles. For instance, the speed of the cell cycle varies enormously, particularly in early embryo development in eukaryotic systems. In these early embryonic cells, no growth occurs, so that each of the two daughter cells derived from a cell division is half the size of the parent cell; the cycle time is very short (8-60 minutes) and no Gl and G2 phases are found so that S and M phases directly alternate with each other (Fig.).

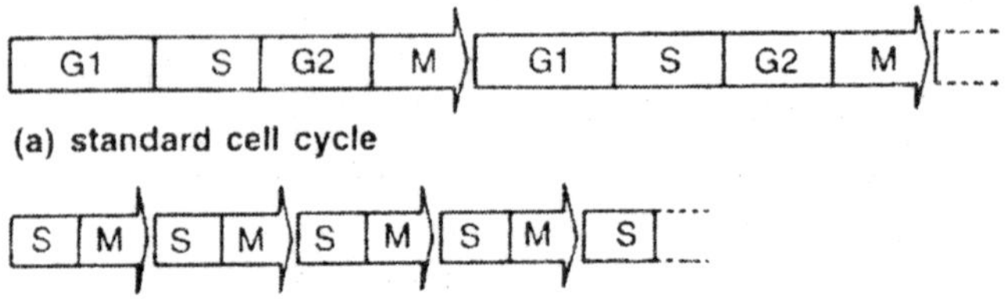

A comparison of the standard cell cycle with the early embryonic cell cycle; note the smaller (half) size and direct alternation of S and M phases (Gl and G2 phases are absent) in the early embryonic cell cycle (redrawn from Alberts et. al., 'Molecular Biology of the Cell', 1994).

These early embryonic cell cycles, in which S and M phases alternate in quick succession without intervening Gl and G2 phases, are the simplest form of cell cycles. Therefore, these embryonic cells have been extensively utilised to understand the mechanisms involved in the regulatory control of the cell cycle progression. In *Drosophila,* cells occupying different positions in the embryo, exhibit G2 phase that differs in length from 30 minutes to 150 minutes. Further, the cell divisions though usually symmetric, may also be asymmetric, as in the production of three polar bodies and one egg from an egg mother cell through a meiotic division. These variations in cell division cycle proved very useful in the study of molecular basis of cell division, both mitosis and meiosis.

Central Cell Cycle Control System: During the last two decades of 20th century, it was shown that there exists a central cell cycle control system, which regulates the orderly progress of events during the cell cycle. An analogy has also been drawn between the cell cycle and an automatic clothes washing machine.

In a washing machine the sequential functions like addition of water and detergent, followed by washing, rinsing and spin drying the clothes have been considered analogous to the essential processes of cell cycle like DNA replication, mitosis and anaphase segregation of chromosomes. In both cases (washing machine and cell cycle), a central control system triggers different processes in a specific, sequence.

Although the control system could operate as a simple clock, allotting a fixed time for each process but the operation of control system is not so simple. Actually, the control system has a feedback device, so that at certain critical points of the cell cycle (also in washing machine) regulation is exercised by feedback from processes that are in progress. For instance, in the washing with the help of a washing machine, there are sensors that monitor the water level and send signals back to the control system to prevent start of next process (*e.g.*, spin drying), before the previous process is completed.

In the cell cycle also, there are devices which ensure that the cell is not driven into mitosis before DNA synthesis is completed or damaged DNA repaired, and it is not driven into anaphase before all chromosomes are aligned on the spindle.

It is apparent from the above analogy that a control system exists, which is distinct from the machinery performing the essential processes. For instance, while there is a machinery involved in DNA synthesis, there is a separate and distinct control system which regulates the entry of the cell into S-phase and later into M-phase (after DNA synthesis is completed).

Such a distinction between a control system and the machinery involved in different processes was recognised rather late Earlier, we thought that each of the essential processes triggers the next process (without any control device), as in a chain of falling dominoes (dominoes are oblong pieces used in a game, where fall of one leads to fall of others in a sequence; Fig.). Thus the cell cycle was described as a set of dependent reactions (with no independent controls) having checkpoints and the theory was described as domino theory.

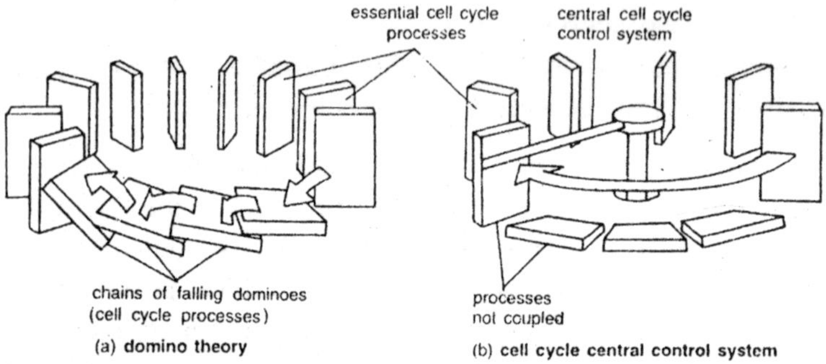

Two alternative concepts of cell cycle control, where slabs represent essential processes of the cell cycle, such as DNA replication, chromosome condensation, spindle formation, etc. (a) domino theory; (b) cyclic control device (as proved in the real cell cycle (redrawn from Alberts et. al., 'Molecular Biology of the Cell', 1994).

According to another theory described as clock theory, the events of cell cycle are assumed to be not directly coupled (an event dependent on the preceding event), but are assumed to occur in succession, regulated by a control system that operates independently of the actual occurrence of these events (Fig. b). The key components of such a central cell-cycle control system have now been identified and have been shown to be distinct from the molecules that perform the essential processes of cell cycle including DNA replication, mitosis and chromosome segregation.

The cell-cycle control system makes use of a set of interacting proteins that induce and coordinate downstream process involved in cell cycle. In this control system there are checkpoints, where brakes and feedback signals can operate. The brakes can stop the cycle at checkpoints and feedback signals can delay progress of the control system itself, so that it will not be able to trigger the next event, before the previous one is completed. The environment also acts on the control system at Gl-S transition (called start in yeast and Gl checkpoint in mammals) or at G2-M transition (called G2 checkpoint).

Cell Cycle Checkpoints

There are also specific surveillance mechanisms that detect mistakes, and induce inhibition of key cell cycle transitions like Gl-S and G2-M transitions in the event of such a mistake (Fig.). There has been rapid progress in the study of these surveillance mechanisms, but only few instances are available where we understand how these mechanisms inhibit key cell cycle transitions in the event of a mistake. An analogy between the mechanisms that check completion of events in cell cycle and the road blocks where travellers are scruitinised, has often been drawn and this actually led to the use of the term 'checkpoints' for these mechanisms.

The word checkpoint suggests the involvement of a place (border) and a process (scrutiny). This assumed duality led to some confusion and the checkpoints have been defined differently by different workers as (i) points in the cell cycle at which processes being monitored are completed; (ii) points in the cell cycle at which transitions are blocked; (iii) biochemical pathways that ensure dependence of one process on another process, which is otherwise biochemically unrelated; mutation in a checkpoint leads to loss of this dependence, so that

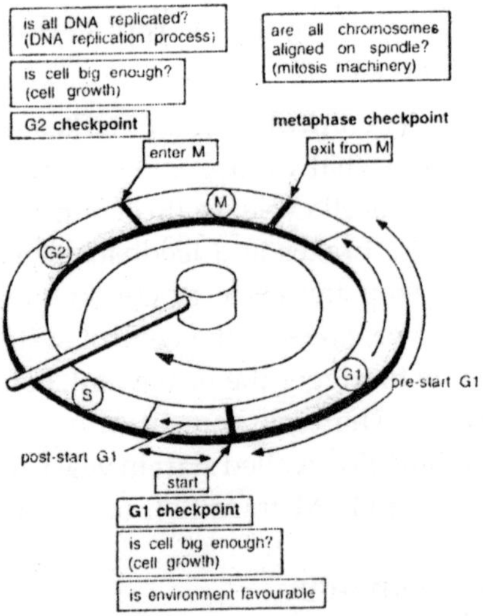

Checkpoint and inputs of regulatory information of the cell cycle control system; the prominent checkpoints are highlighted, but other checkpoints are also found as discussed in the text, (redrawn from Alberts et. al., 'Molecular Biology of the Cell', 1994).

checkpoints are inhibitory pathways; (iv) controls that ensure progress of cell division in a specific order of the cell cycle events or transitions. Checkpoints are also regarded to be signal transduction pathways involving initiating signals, sensors, transducers and effectors.

The checkpoints as above make use of CDKs *(cyclin dependent kinase-cyclin* complexes) to exercise controls during the cell cycle. CDKs described later in this chapter, are actually used by cells to facilitate progressions through cell cycle transitions. Inhibition of these CDKs leads to cell cycle arrest.

These inhibition pathways are actually the checkpoints. Many checkpoint pathways have been identified primarily through the analysis of *cdc/CDC* mutants in yeasts and include the checkpoints, that: (i) sense mating partners, (ii) coordinate cell size and cell cycle progression; (iii) inhibit mitosis while in Gl; (iv) make nuclear division dependent upon budding; (v) restrict DNA replication to once per cycle; (vi) make DNA synthesis dependent upon Gl cyclins; (vii) cause delay in entry from G2 into M phase and from Gl into S phase in the event of DNA damage; (viii) cause delay in separation of chromatids at anaphase, until all the chromosomes are duly aligned on the spindle.

Feedback Controls and Inhibitory Signals: During the progression of different stages in the cell cycle, feedback controls ensure that the cell cycle does not proceed to the next step before the preceding step is duly completed, because such a premature entry into next step will be disastrous for the cell. Feedback control in other words means that a particular stage of cell cycle will keep track whether or not the preceding stage is completed and will not start, unless this previous stage gets completed. For instance, there are mechanisms which ensure that the cell is not driven into mitosis before DNA synthesis is completed and that it is not driven into anaphase before all the chromosomes are aligned on" the spindle. These mechanisms are facilitated by feedback controls, which operate at checkpoints meant for arresting the cell cycle progression before a process is completed.

Following are some examples of feedback controls: (i) A feedback control has been detected, which delays mitosis until DNA replication is complete. This is demonstrated by experiments, in which, if DNA synthesis is blocked (*e.g.*, by amphidocolin or by hydroxyurea), the cells halt at S-phase and will not progress to mitosis. This is due to a feedback control on the start of mitosis, which can be destroyed by substances like caffeine, so that cells enter into mitosis even before DNA synthesis is complete, (ii) A feedback control also exists which detects DNA damage and does not allow entry of cell into mitosis until the damage is repaired.

The gene *rad9* in yeast has been shown to code for an essential component of this feedback control. Mutants lacking *rad9* although repair DNA damage, but can not delay mitotic entry of G2 cells, so that the cells enter mitosis with damaged chromosomes. Similarly in mammals, protein p53 causes delay in the entry of cells with damaged DNA into S-phase, so that the cells stay in Gl. Mutation in *p53* gene, therefore causes cancer, due to increase in frequency of cancer promoting genetic alterations.

Cyclin Dependent Kinases (Cdks) and Cyclins (Cell Cycle's Engine): On the basis of results of studies on yeast, fruitfly, frog and mammals, it has now been established that the eukaryotic cell cycle in majority of eukaryotes, is governed by two major types of proteins (i) cyclin dependent kinases *(Cdks)* and (ii) cyclins (so named, because their abundance differs through the cell cycle). Cdk (kinase subunit) associates with cyclin (regulatory subunit) to form a Cdk-cyclin complex, to which we like to give the symbol CDK. (There seems to be confusion in the literature about the usage of symbols Cdk and CDK, each being used by different workers either for cyclin dependent kinase alone or for cyclin dependent kinase-cyclin complex. In this chapter we like to use Cdk for the cyclin dependent kinase alone and CDK for the Cdk-cyclin complex). Recognising the pre-eminent role of Cdk-cyclin complex in cell division, this complex has also been described as cell cycle's engine. Although originally Cdk-cyclin complexes were recognised as cell cycle regulatory proteins, they are now also known to control functions other than regulating the cell cycle, like transcription and cell metabolism.

The Cdk subunit is inactive as a protein kinase without the cyclin subunit, which confers basal kinase activity to the Cdk due to conformational changes caused by the binding of the cyclin. However a mere association of cyclin and Cdk is not sufficient to confer kinase activity to Cdk, since its activity is controlled *firstly,* through a programme of activating and inhibitory phosphorylation events and *secondly,* through the association with different classes of regulatory molecules

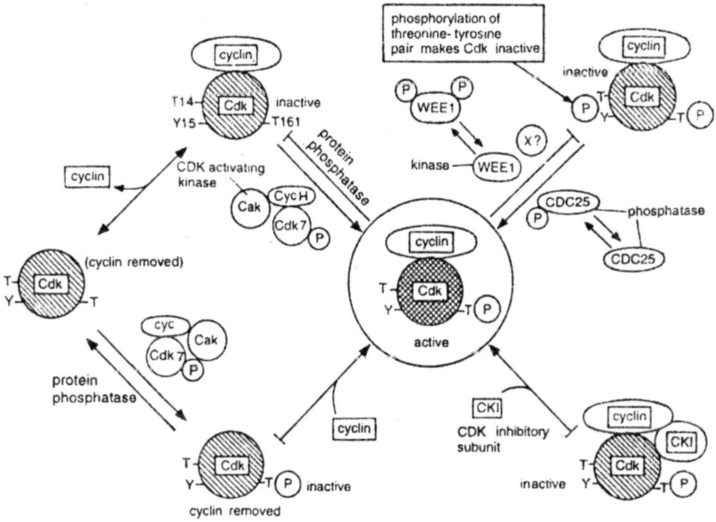

Different stimulatory (→) and inhibitory (—1) steps involving reversible phosphorylation of Cdk-cyclin (CDK) complexes.

including cyclins and inhibitors. Both Cdk and cyclin have one or more amino acid residues (threonine or tyrosine), which can be phosphorylated and dephosphorylated (reversible phosphorylation). For instance, in the Cdk subunit of CDK, phosphorylation of a threonine residue (thr-167 in cdc2p of fission yeast, thr-169 in CDC28p of budding yeast and thr-161 in p33/p34 of humans) by Cdk activating kinase (Cak) and dephosphorylation of another residue due to a phosphatase, results in full activity of Cdk.

Binding of cyclin subunit also modulates substrate specificity of the kinase. A number of Cdks (Cdkl to Cdk7) are now known, which include Cdkl (corresponds cdc2 or $p34^{cdc2}$ in fission yeast and CDC28 in budding yeast) in yeasts, Cdkl and Cdk2 in majority of animals and Cdkl, Cdk2, Cdk3, Cdk4 and Cdk6 in mammals. Similarly, following three types of cyclins are known: (i) mitotic cyclins (cyclin B; also called cdcl3p in fission yeast and CLBs= CLB1-6 in budding yeast) found during M phase; (ii) S-phase cyclins (cyclin A), found during S-phase and (iii) Gl cyclins (called cig1 and cig2 in fission yeast; CLN1, CLN2 and CLN3 in budding yeast and cyclins C, D, E and F in vertebrates) found during Gl phase.

Both in budding and fission yeasts, S and M phases are induced by a solitary Cdkl (CDC28 in budding yeast and cdc2 in fission yeast) which is associated with different cyclins (one at a time), specific for S-phase and M-phase. In animal cells at least two different Cdk proteins are needed one for each of the two major checkpoints (Gl and G2 checkpoints). S-phase is induced by Cdk2 complexed with S-phase cyclins (E or A types) and M-phase is induced by Cdkl complexed with M phase cyclins, *i.e.*, A and B types (Table). In mammals there are additional kinases like Cdk4, Cdk6 that are specialised for different transitions.

Cdks and Cyclins Involved in G2/M and G1/S Transitions of Cell Cycle

	G2/M phase		*G1/S phase*	
	Cdk	*Cyclin*	*Cdk*	*Cyclin*
S. pombe (fission yeast)	cdc2 (Cdkl)	cdc 13 (A like)	cdc2 (Cdkl)	cigl, cig2
S. *cerevisiae* (budding yeast)	CDC28 (Cdkl)	CLB1-4 (B like) (associates after START)	CDC28 (Cdkl)	CLN1-3
Mammal/frog	Cdc 2 (Cdkl)	A, Bl, B2	Cdk2 (p33), Cdk4, Cdk6	A, Dl, D2, D3, E

CDKs and Cyclins in Fission Yeast: In fission yeast, a single Cdk (Cdkl) encoded by *cdc2* (its corresponding gene in budding yeast is *CDC28),* and three cyclins encoded by *cdc13, cigl* and *cigl* are now known to control cell-cycle progression. Cyclin cdcl3, also called cyclin A, (and to a minor extent also cigl protein) activates Cdk1 or cdc2 protein ($p34^{cdc2}$, molecular weight, 34kD) at the time of onset of mitosis (G2-M transition); later, after completion of mitosis, the degradation of cdc13 (molecular weight, 45kD) leads to inactivation of this Cdkl ($p34^{cdc2}$). This is a prerequisite for mitotic exit. Although cigl might make a minor contribution to activation of cdc2, but it is not essential for onset of mitosis.

Recently cig2 has been shown to be a major partner of cdc2 in Gl phase (in G2 phase, for entry into M phase, the major partner of cdc2 is the product of gene *cdc13).* The quantity of cig2 and the associated kinase activity are periodic, reaching a peak around Gl-S transition. However, cig2 is not essential for the initiation of S-phase, and the absence of cig2 causes only delay in Gl-S transition. It is also known that in the absence of cig2, the cyclin cdc13 (earlier thought to be acting exclusively as mitotic cyclin) is involved in the cyclin dependent kinase activity of-cdc2, even in S-phase.

It has been observed, that the cdcl3 level begins to increase only after initiation of S phase. In mutants lacking cig2 (cig2 Δ), S phase is delayed; in mutants lacking both cig2 and cdcl3 (cig2 Δ cdcl3 Δ), S phase is severely compromised and in mutants lacking all the three cyclins, cigl, cig2 and cdcl3 (cigl Δ cig2 Δ cdcl3 Δ), the S phase is completely blocked. This suggests that actually all the three cyclins contribute to CDK activity of cdc2 during S phase.

However, in mutants lacking both cigl and cig2, orderly onset of S phase and mitosis can take place, suggesting that quantitative differences in cdcl3 dependent kinase activity of cdc2, rather than qualitative difference, may regulate onset of

S phase and mitosis. Thus cdcl3 can fulfil three different functions in association with cdc2: (i) it is essential for the onset of mitosis; (ii) it prevents re-replication in G2 and (iii) it compensates for cig2 as the major Gl cyclin in mutants lacking cig2 (cig2 Δ).

There are two possible models to explain how cdc2-cdcl3 can bring about the onset of both S phase and M phase (mitosis), (i) In the first model, the activity of cdc2-cdcl3 CDK is modified by different modifers at Gl and G2 phases, (ii) In the second model, cdc2 kinase activity in cdc2-cdcl3 association differs quantitatively at Gl and G2 phases.

The onset of S phase requires a lower threshold relative to that required for the onset of M phase (Fig.). The CDKs, which are Cdk-cyclin complexes, are both positively and negatively regulated by phosphorylation. Cdks are further regulated by binding of inhibitors (CKIs) and other proteins such as Sucl (Cksl).

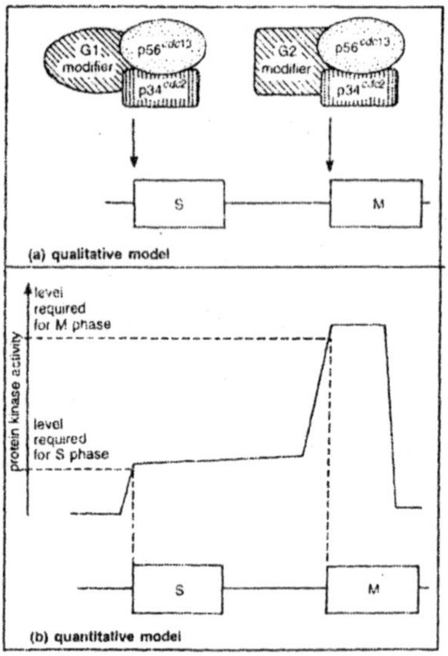

Two models to explain the role of Cdc2-cdcl3 complex in the onset of S phase and M phase.

CDKs are not the only conserved factors, changes in the activity of which promote S and M phase. In late Gl, Cdk7 kinase is activated by Dbf4 (Cdk7 is therefore called Dbf4 dependent kinase or Dbk) and in late G2, Cdk5 is activated by Polo (Polo/Cdc5 kinase). The coordinated activity of cdc2 and cdcl3 is regulated by two additional genes *cdc25* (stimulates entry into mitosis), and *weel* (inhibits entry into mitosis), which act antagonistically to control and regulate the entry of cell into mitosis. Another gene *niml* exercises a negative control on *weel* (Fig.).

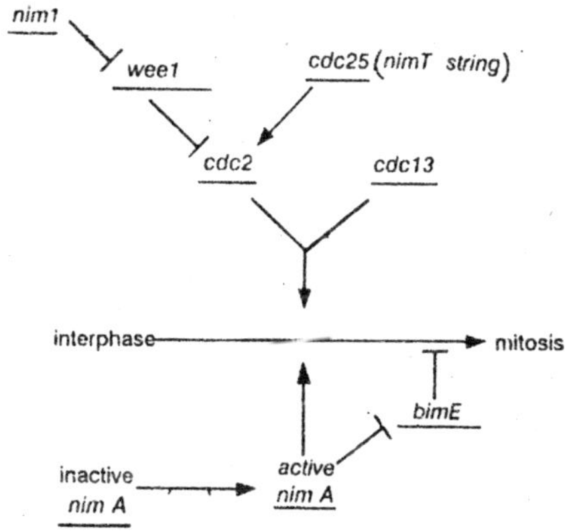

A model for induction of mitosis in the fission yeast. Gene products are shown as stimulating (→) or inhibiting (—I) the activity of other gene products. The cdc2 and cdcli gene products are shown acting in conceil to induce mitosis.

Both *niml* and *weel* are believed to produce kinases (kinases cause phosphorylation) and *cdc25* produces a phosphatase (phosphatases cause dephosphorylation), which removes phosphate from a tyrosine residue (tyr-15) of $p34^{cdc2}$. Therefore, these genes act through regulation of protein phosphorylation and dephosphorylation. An increase in the ratio of activities of two genes, namely that of *cdc25* to *weel,* increases the cell size required for entry into mitosis, while a decrease in this ratio leads to decrease in this critical cell size. The overexpression of *cdc25* in a strain, mutant for *weel,* causes premature entry into mitosis resulting into lethality. It has also been shown that a *Drosophila* gene named *string* (required for later embryonic cell cycles) is homologous to *cdc25* and produces Cds^{string}. A model for the pathway that leads to the induction of mitosis has been constructed from genetic analysis of the above mutants in fission yeast and is presented in Figure.

CDKs and Cyclin in Budding Yeast: In budding yeast, although five Cdks (CDC28, PHO85, KIN28, SRB10 and CTK1) are known, but only one (CDC28) is involved in cell division cycle (Table). The other Cdks contribute to cell cycle progression through regulation of gene expression and cell metabolism. Cdks have a conserved core sequence of about 300 amino acids. This core sequence represents the catalytic site, which is though homologous to the catalytic site of other cyclic AMP dependent kinases (*e.g.*, PKA), but differs in minor details reflecting differences in their regulation. Cdks also contain several α -helices, one of them (α_1) containing a PSTAIRE sequence motif characteristic of the Cdk family (in PSTAIRE, each letter means an individual amino acid; for single letter abbreviations of amino acids. This sequence represents a domain that is conserved between yeast and human cdc2. Cdks are sometime also named after their amino acid sequence in the PSTAIRE region. For instance, earlier Cdk5 was known as PSSALRE and Cdk6 was known as PLSTIRE.

There are also as many as 22 cyclins known in budding yeast; each binds to one of the five Cdks listed above. Nine of these cyclins are known to activate CDC28, the key Cdk in cell cycle progress (Table). Cyclins vary in their molecular weight from 30kD to 45kD. All cyclins have a region of homology, 100 amino acids in length and called 'cyclin box' made up of a motif called 'cyclin fold". This cyclin box clamps and surrounds the middle part of the PSTAIRE helix and forms the centerpiece of the cyclin-Cdk specificity. The activation of Cdk, in association with cyclin is actually due to conformational change in PSTAIRE helix. The association of cyclin with Cdk also exposes amino acid residues, that are the substrate for Dhosphorvlation by Cdk.

Cdks and their Cyclins in Budding Yeast (S. Cerevisiae)

Cdk	*Cyclins*	*Cdk-cydin function*
CDC28	CLN1, CLN2, CLN3	START (Sic 1p proteolysis, inhibition of CLB proteolysis, activation of Gl transcription)
	CLB5, CLB6	DNA replication
	CLB1 to CLB4	Mitosis, spindle assembly.
PHO85	PCL1	Needed for START in the absence of CLN1 and CLN2
	CLG1, PCL5, PCL9	Unknown
	PHO80	Regulates transcription factor PHO4p
	PCL6, PCL17	Unknown
	PCL8, PCL10	Glycogen synthase kinase
KIN28	CCL1	Transcription (CTD kinase)
SRB10	SRB11	Transcription (CTD kinase)
CTK1	CTK2	Transcription (CTD kinase)

In budding yeast, a single Cdk (Cdkl=CDC28) associates with three cyclins (CLN1, CLN2, CLN3) for transitions from Gl to S-phase. The same Cdk (CDC28) also associates with B-type cyclins (CLBl-CLB4p) for progression after start, the cyclin CLB2 being the most important for the transition from G2 to M phase. Further, in budding yeast, the transcription of two cyclin genes *(CLN1, CLN2)* requires two additional genes *SWI4* and *SWI6* (responsible for gene switching at the mating type locus). The products of these two genes are components of α transcription factor. (In budding yeast 'α' factor and 'a' factor are two mating type factors and a type factor inhibits SWI4 and SWI6 to bring about arrest of cell division to facilitate conjugation.

All the three *CLN* genes *(CLN1, CLN2, CLN3)* need to be

inactivated to block the passage through START, *i.e.*, from Gl to S-phase. The *CLN* genes are thus functionally redundant, because even one of the three is, adequate to allow progression from Gl to S-phase and mutation in one or even two of these genes fail to block the cell cycle. Similarly, mutation in any one of the *CLB* genes fails to block cell division, but the loss of both *CLB1* and *CLB2* is lethal, and loss of *CLB1* alone prevents cell's exit from mitosis.

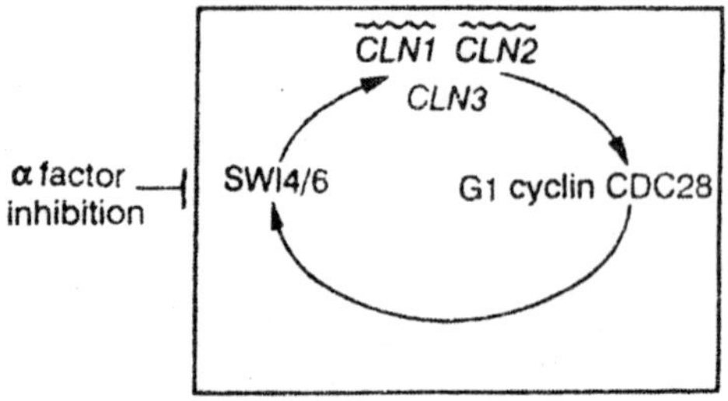

Positive feedback loop involving budding yeast Gl cyclins. Wavy lines show the genes thought to be activated at the transcriptional level by SW14/6; α factor is an inhibitor of the feedback loop and behaves as a negative growth factor for yeast.

The above feature of redundancy observed in *CLN* and *CLB* genes is also found elsewhere in cell cycle genes. For instance, G2/M transition in fission yeast is inhibited by redundant kinases weel and mikl and redundant genes encoding phosphatases (cdc25, pyp3) have also been reported. In each case, deletion of one gene gives a cyclic phenotype, but deletion of all redundant genes of a group is lethal. This suggests that redundant members of a group may have overlapping, rather than identical functions.

Cyclins in Mammalian Cells: In contrast to yeasts, where a single Cdk is known to control the cell cycle progression, in mammalian cells, atleast two and under special situations (*e.g.* cell growth) more than two Cdks are used. Cdkl (cdc2 protein) complexed with cyclin B is used for passage through mitosis or M-phase and Cdk2 complexed with cyclin A is needed to activate the DNA replication machinery (Fig.). Cdk4 and Cdk6, complexed with cyclin D, on the other hand, are involved in cell growth (particularly after exit from a quiescent or GO phase), and are, therefore, not produced periodically during the cell cycle (unlike Cdkl and Cdk2) .

Binding of cyclin subunit also modulates the substrate specificity of the kinase, *i.e.*, Cdk. These substrates may include the following: (i) retinoblastoma protein (Rb), phosphorylated by Cdk4-cyclin D; (ii) pl07, E2F and replication protein-A, phosphorylated by Cdk2-cyclin A and (iii) histone H1, phosphorylated by Cdkl-cyclin B.

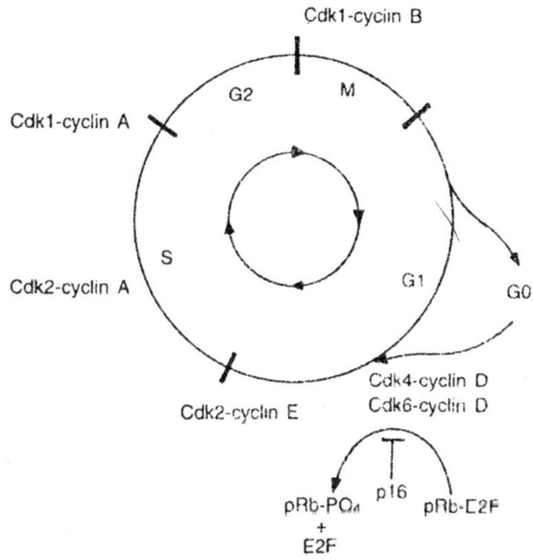

An outline of cell cycle in a mammalian cell, showing the roles of a number of cyclinsA,B, D,E) in the form of Cdk-cyclin complexes, which facilitate passage through different phases of the cell cycle.

The activation of Cdkl-cyclin B complex also needs phosphatase CDC25 in late G2 to bring about dephosphorylation needed for activation of Cdkl. The complex Cdk2-cyclinA has also been studied in some detail by X-ray crystallography (reported in 1995), to explain the structural basis of regulation of Cdks. It has been shown that cyclin A

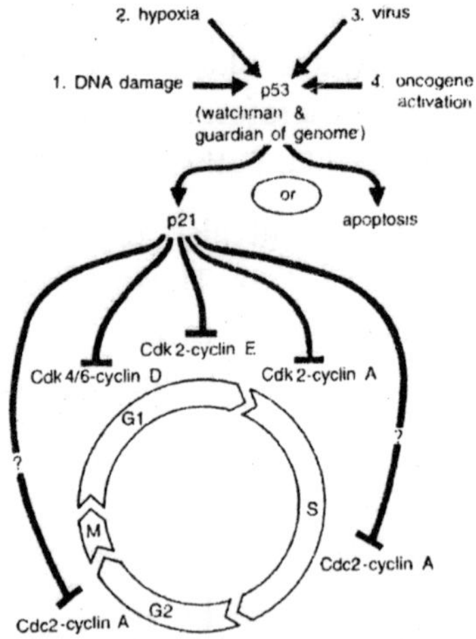

A model showing the roles of p53 and p21 in regulating the different phases of cell cycle in a mammalian cell.

modifies Cdk2 structure by reorienting a glutamic acid residue into the catalytic cleft and moving away the regulatory loop, thus blocking the access of a substrate for phosphorylation. Further, the Cdk2-cyclin A needs to be phosphorylated at threonine-160 for full activation. Binding of p27 with the complex Cdk2-cyclin A physically blocks the active site. There are also other non-cyclin proteins that play a major role in cell cycle regulation in the mammalian cells. Following are some examples:

(i) p53 (product of a tumour suppression gene) is a strong activator of transcription and responds to DNA damage or to conditions unfavourable for DNA replication; in its turn it activates a number of genes including the gene *p21;* the protein p21 is a Cdk-cyclin inhibitor, and therefore arrests the progression of cell cycle, thus permitting time for DNA repair (Fig.);

(ii) E2F (a transcription factor required for expression of adenovirus E2 gene) also plays a predominant role in cell cycle regulation; it also interacts with other proteins like p53, Rb, pl07 and pl30.

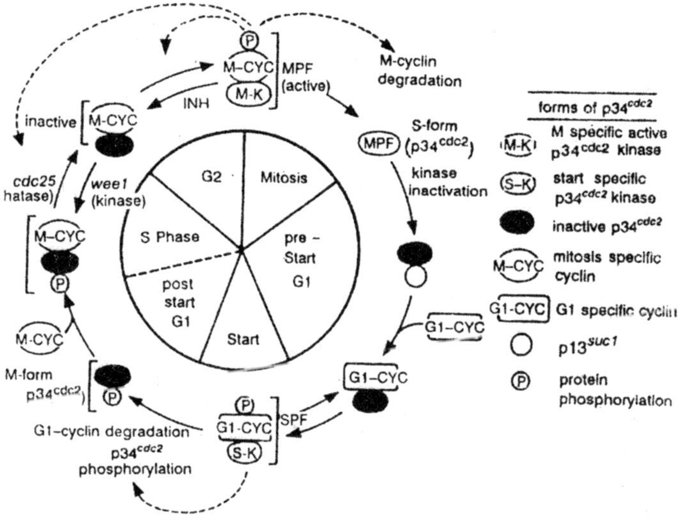

A model of the cycle of cdc2 gene product ($p34^{cdc2}$) during the cell cycle in fission yeast.(Note that $p34^{lydc2}$ molecule lacks kinase activity during most of the cell cycle, but becomes active as MPF at mitosis and SPF at start as a result of association with M cyclins and Gl cyclins respectively; active forms can also stimulate their own activation and/or inactivation (→); the dashed line between post-start Gl and S phases indicates that no change in $p34^{cdc2}$ occurs during onset of DNA synthesis.

Association of two Alternative Forms of Cdk (M and S forms) with M Cyclins and Gl Cyclins: The Cdkl ($p34^{cdc2}$ in fission yeast and CDC28 in budding yeast) in yeasts is believed to exist in two forms (M-form and S-form), which differ from each other due to post-translational modifications of this protein. We will discuss this alternation of M and S forms for fission yeast, but the corresponding M and S forms will be available in budding yeast also.

In fission yeast, in combination with mitotic (M) cyclin (cdcl3), Cdkl ($p34^{cdc2}$) can form active protein kinase, known as M-phase promoting factor or MPF, which induces the events of mitosis. (MPF was earlier described as maturation promoting factor, by biochemists). Later, during the passage through mitosis, M-form of $p34^{cdc2}$ changes to S-form, which combines with Gl cyclins to form start promoting factor (SPF). This SPF catalyzes passage through 'start' (an event that commits the cell to initiate DNA replication). At some point, after start, but before completion of S-phase, S-form of Cdkl ($p34^{cdc2}$) again changes to M-form, which, in association of M cyclins (cdc 13), gives active MPF. The formation of active MPF guarantees completion of S-phase of cell cycle. Thus the alternation of replication (S phase) and segregation (M phase) is actually brought about by alternating activation of Cdkl component of the SPF and MPF (Figs.).

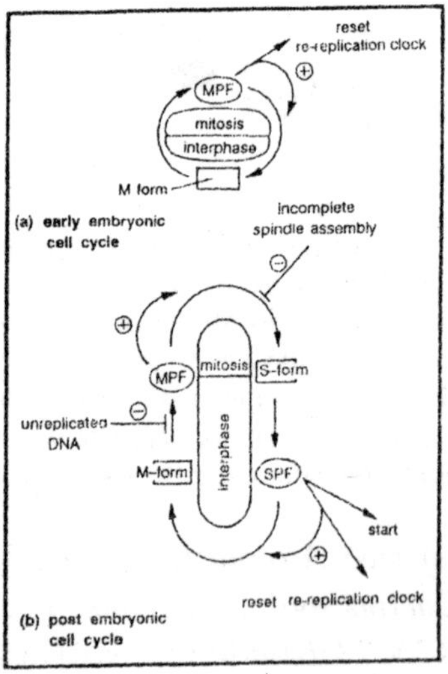

Models of the early embryonic and post embryonic cell cycles: (a) In the early embryonic cell cycle only, $p34^{cdc2}$ is present in only one form (M form); block to re-replication of DNA is removed by activation of MPF. (b) In post-embryonic cell cycle, $p34^{cdc2}$ exists in two forms (M form and S form) giving MPF and SPF. Feedback controls regulate the activation and inactivation of MPF to ensure that mitosis does not begin till DNA replication is complete, and anaphase does not begin until assembly of spindle is finished.

How is this alternation of activities actually brought about? One hypothesis suggests that Gl cyclins and M cyclins are synthesized at different points in the cell cycle. However, it has also been shown that modified M cyclins can also perform the function of Gl cyclins. Another gene product required for conversion of M-form of Cdkl into its S-form, is $pl3^{suc1}$

(also called Suc1, and is the product of fission yeast gene *suc1)*, which is known to bind to Cdkl component of MPF.

Reversible Phosphorylation of CDKs, and CDK Activation Kinases (Caks): During the cell division cycle, activation of CDKs (Cdk/cyclin complexes) is regulated by reversible phosphorylation due to kinase (for phosphorylation) and phosphatase (for dephosphorylation) activities of certain proteins. For instance, in fission yeast activities of genes *cdc2* (gene product is a Cdk) and *cdcl3* (gene product is a cyclin) are regulated by atleast three other genes including two genes *(niml* and *weel)* producing kinases and one gene *(cdc25)* producing a phosphatase.

The genes *cdc25* and *weel* work antagonistically and *niml* exercises a negative control on *weel* (Fig.). While, *cdc2* producing Cdkl (a kinase) is responsible for phosphorylation of cyclin proteins, *weel* is responsible for the phosphorylation of Cdkl. The gene *cdc25*, on the other hand, is responsible for dephosphorylation of Cdkl. Such kinases and phosphatases regulating cell division cycle have also been discovered in other organisms. For instance, in *Aspergillus*, product of *nimT* (homologue of *cdc25* in fission yeast and *MIH1* in budding yeast) is a phosphatase and that of *nimA* is a kinase *(nim* mutant = never in mitosis, meaning that it can not enter mitosis after DNA synthesis). The gene *nimA* actually inhibits the activity of yet another gene in *Aspergillus*, namely *bimE (bimE* mutant = blocked in mitosis, meaning that it can not exit from mitosis; Fig.

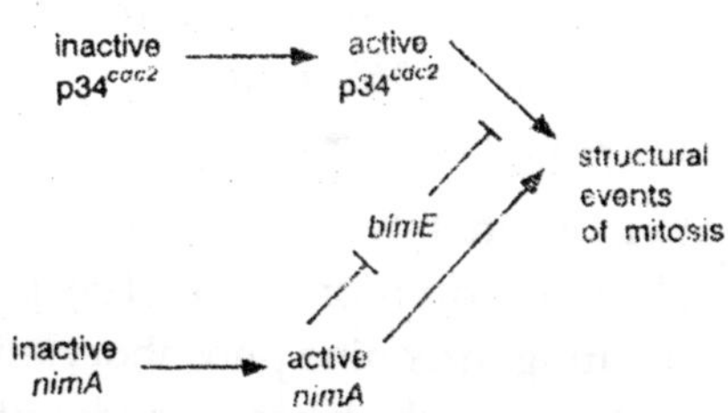

Interactions between $p34^{cdc2}$, nim A and bim E and the induction of mitosis (—I indicates inhibitory interactions).

The phosphorylation of Cdkl ($p34^{cdc2}$) in fission yeast involves tyrosine and threonine residues. After passing through 'start', the cells synthesize mitotic cyclins (cyclin B), which accumulate and bind to Cdkl ($p34^{cdc2}$). This complex is initially inactive, due to associated phosphorylation of tyrosine 15 (tyr-15) of Cdkl (tyr-15 phosphorylation inhibits kinase activity). This inactive complex undergoes further phosphorylation at threonine 167 (thr-167), which is necessary for MPF activity, but is not sufficient to overcome the inhibitory effect of tyrosine phosphorylation.

Subsequent removal of tyrosine phosphate from Cdkl during G2 activates MPF and leads to induction of mitosis (M phase). In fission yeast, tyrosine kinase is the product of the gene *weel*, whereas phosphatase is the product of the gene *cdc25*. Active MPF activates tyr-phosphatase and inhibits tyr-kinase. This leads to entry into mitosis. MPF induces chromosome condensation, nuclear envelope breakdown and assembly of spindle. MPF also activates enzymes that conjugate ubiquitin to cyclin leading to ubiquitin dependent cyclin degradation (with the help of proteasome; see later), which renders MPF inactive. Cyclin degradation and MPF inactivation lead to chromosome segregation, chromosome decondensation, nuclear reformation and cytokinesis.

Based on the above discussion, we may summarise that in budding yeast, phosphorylation of threonine-169 in CDC28, and in fission yeast phosphorylation of threonine-167 in cdc2 is required for G2/M transition and its dephosphorylation is required for Gl/S transition. Similarly, reversible phosphorylation of threonine 161 in human Cdk is needed for the above two checkpoints.

Thus it is obvious, that tyrosine and threonine kinase activities are vital in cell division cycle. The protein kinase responsible for activating threonine phosphorylation is named Cak (Cdk activating kinase), which has been identified in higher eukaryotes,. The Cak is itself a Cdk, called Cdk7 or MO15

(Cdk7 is a Dbk = Dbf4 dependent kinase), which associates with cyclin H to bring about threonine phosphorylation. This Cak protein is also a component of transcription factor TFIIH, phosphorylating C-terminal repeat domain (CTD) of the largest subunit of RNA polymerase II. Cdk7/cyclinH complex, therefore has a role both in transcription and cell division progression. In budding yeast, however, CTD kinase and Cak are encoded in different genes. In budding yeast Cakl has been identified, which phosphorylates and activates CDC28/CLB2. Cakl has been shown to be essential for G2 to M U'ansition as well as for Gl to S transition (due to activation of CDC28).

Cdk inhibitors (CKIs) and Sucl (Cksl): The activity of Cdk is also regulated by binding to inhibitors called cyclin dependent kinase inhibitors (CKIs) and by other proteins like Sucl (Cksl). It has been shown that cell growth is also controlled or inhibited by the products of tumour suppressor genes like *RB* (retinoblastoma), which maintain the cells at Gl or GO (G zero). Several of the growth inhibiting signals, including the growth inhibitory factor TGF-β act through inhibitors of Cdk-cyclin complexes which are described as cyclin dependent kinase inhibitors (CKIs). These CKIs (*e.g.* Sicl, Farl, Runıl, p21, p27, p57, pl6, pl5, pl8, pl9) are found associated with CDKs thus inactivating them as observed in quiescent cells at GO state. Several of these CKIs have been characterised and named according to their molecular sizes; *e.g.* pl5/pl6 (ink4), p21(cip/WATl) and p27(kipl).

The proteins pl5/pl6 are coded by two adjacent genes and pl6 binds specifically to Cdk4 and Cdk6, suggesting a connection with G0/G1 transition. The protein p21 is a universal Cdk inhibitor and binds with Cdk2, Cdk4 and Cdk6, suggesting that it inhibits progression through all stages of Gl/S. The protein p27 is a sequence that is partly related to p21 and binds promiscuously to all Cdk-cyclin complexes. Overexpression of p27 blocks progression through S phase, and its poor expression leads to poor survival of patients suffering with breast or colorectal cancers. A protein, p38 (encoded by *Jabl)* causes degradation of p27. Both p21 and p27 bind and render the Cdk-cyclin complex incapable of being activated through phosphorylation by Cak. Another cyclin dependent kinase inhibitor is rum 1, which also causes re-replication and results in concomitant accumulation of cdcl8p.

Interaction of cdc6p, cdcl8p and Ruml with CDKs: The proteins cdc6p in budding yeast and cdcl8p in fission yeast are important proteins that remain associated with CDK and influence the cell cycle through their effect on DNA replication. As discussed earlier, cdc6p and origin recognition complex (ORC) nucleate MCM proteins to chromatin and thus help in DNA replication, since MCM proteins are absolutely necessary for the replication to proceed further (Fig.).

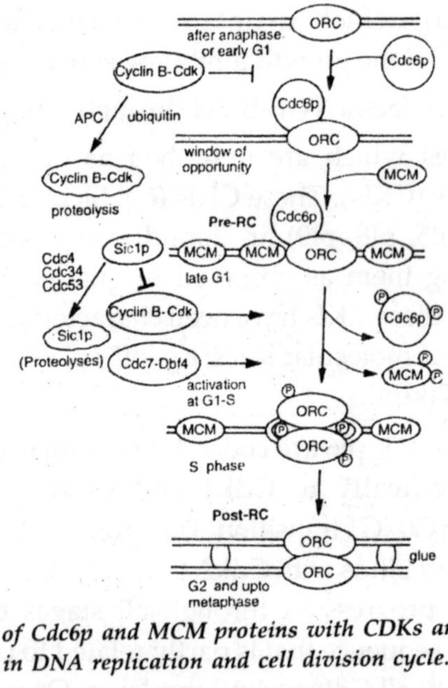

Interaction of Cdc6p and MCM proteins with CDKs and their role in DNA replication and cell division cycle.

Similarly cdcl8p in fission yeast plays an important role in DNA replication and is required for (i) entry into S-phase

(ii) limiting DNA replication to once per cell cycle and (iii) coupling of mitosis to completion of S phase. This protein (cdcl8p) is highly unstable and is expressed only once per cell cycle, *i.e.*, at the Gl/S boundary.

As soon as the cell crosses START, cdcl8p is produced. Its absence blocks entry into S phase and uncouples dependence of mitosis on completion of S phase. Its overexpression allows multiple cycles of DNA replication to occur without mitosis. It has been shown that cdc18p interacts with CDK complex and that CDK can phosphorylate cdcl8p thus rendering cdcl8p inactive and ready for proteolytic degradation. When CDK (cdc2/cdcl3) is inactive, cdcl8p is active and *vice-versa*, so that as soon as cdc2/cdcl3 becomes active and allows entry into M-phase, cdcl8p becomes inactive and DNA re-replication is avoided.

Activity of cdc2/cdcl3 (CDK) is also influenced by another protein ruml (replication uncoupled from mitosis), which regulates progression through Gl phase and thus controls entry into S-phase. Overexpression of ruml, like cdcl8p, also allows multiple rounds of replication to occur (endoreduplication leading to origin of polyploid cells), so that the cell fails to enter mitosis. When the gene *ruml* is deleted, the cells enter mitosis prematurely suggesting that ruml is a CDK inhibitor at M-phase. In other words deletion of *rum1* allows the cells to undergo two successive mitoses without an intervening pre-start G-l phase. While ruml inactivates M phase CDK (cdc2/cdcl3), it simultaneously activates cdcl8p by dephosphorylating it.

cdc18 —CDK (cdc2/cdc13)→ cdc18-p —ruml→ cdc18
(active) (initiates S-phase) | (inactive) (M-phase initiated) | (active) (M-phase inhibited & S-phase initiated)

Dependence of Mitosis on DNA Replication and DNA Repair: For successful progression of cell cycle, it is necessary that DNA replication is completed before the cell enters mitosis. Similarly, if there is DNA damage, it is necessary that this damaged DNA is repaired before the cell cycle progresses any further. In the cell, there are DNA damage and DNA replication checkpoints, which will perform the following functions: (i) sense mating partners; (ii) coordinate cell size and cell cycle progression; (iii) inhibit mitosis while cells are in Gl ; (iv) make DNA replication dependent upon budding; (v) restrict DNA replication to one per cell and (vi) make DNA synthesis dependent upon Gl cyclins. The cells, which suffer either DNA damage or/and a block in DNA replication, exhibit following responses: (i) cell cycle arrest in Gl, S and G2; (ii) slowing of DNA replication and (iii) increase in transcription of genes meant for DNA repair and DNA replication. These responses involve signals, sensors, transducers and effectors.

DNA replication checkpoint-the licensing concept. Important information on the control of DNA replication came from experiments involving cell fusion, among human HeLa cells that were synchronized at various stages of cell cycle and were marked (Fig.). For example, when Gl cells were fused with S phase cells, Gl derived nuclei immediately initiated DNA replication, much earlier than in the Gl cells not so fused. But G2 cells could not activate Gl nuclei. Similarly no DNA replication could be initiated in G2 nuclei when G2 cells were fused with S phase cells. These cell fusion experiments revealed following three important phenomena: (i) only chromosomes from Gl cells are competent to initiate DNA replication; (ii) S phase cells, but not cells in Gl or G2 contain an activator of initiation of DNA replication that can work on competent Gl state; (iii) G2 nuclei do not re-replicate DNA until they pass through mitosis. The current research is, therefore, addressed to the following questions, (i) how is competent state established? (ii) what is the nature of activator in S-phase cells?; (iii) what prevents G2 nuclei from re-replicating? and (iv) how the competent state is erased during mitosis?

On the basis of above cell fusion studies and other studies, a 'licensing factor' model has been proposed, according to which, after the disassembly of nuclear envelope, the replication licensing factors (RLFs) bind to chromatin. This makes the chromosomes competent to replicate. Once the replication is complete, these RLFs would be destroyed thus preventing further round of DNA replication. Two activities, RLF-M and RLF-B have been identified that are required to modify or 'license' chromatin for undergoing replication. A family of proteins, called MCM (minichromosome, *i.e.*, plasmid maintenance) proteins has also been identified in budding yeast, which contributes to the competent state of replication in Gl. These MCM proteins are needed for the maintenance of some plasmids and were identified in some mutants of budding yeast, exhibiting preferential loss of two plasmids.

Atleast six MCM proteins have been identified-MCM2, MCM3, MCM4 (CDC54), MCM5 (CDC46), MCM6, MCM7 (CDC47). The MCM proteins have also been implicated in limiting DNA replication to one per cycle. RLF-M has been shown to contain some MCM proteins, but identity of RLF-B has not been determined. The nucleation of MCM proteins is facilitated by the protein cdc6p/cdc 18p.

In budding yeast, RAD9 specifies a component of the above control system. A number of temperature sensitive mutants defective in DNA synthesis machinery have been isolated, which do not normally undergo mitosis at the restrictive temperature independent of the DNA synthesis.

These mutations (or cells damaged by irradiation) involve fission yeast genes *cdcl7* (DNA polymerase I), *cdc9* (DNA polymerase II) and *cdc2* (DNA polymerase III), the corresponding genes in budding yeast being *POL1, POL2* and *POL3.* However, this dependence of mitosis on DNA synthesis in these mutants is relieved by a complete deficiency of *RAD9.*

In other words, if these *cdc* or *POL* mutants are combined with *RAD9* gene defect, then the cells continue into the next cell cycle at the restrictive temperature. It means that *RAD9* may inhibit mitosis in these mutants and the mutation in *RAD9* releases this negative control, thus permitting mitosis to be completed in these mutants even when DNA synthesis is interrupted.

It is speculated that *RAD9* gene product may interact with MPF or other components known to play essential roles in the initiation of mitosis. In budding yeast *(S. cerevisiae)*, expression of 17 genes is required for DNA synthesis, and their expression is co-regulated due to presence of a common upstream regulatory sequence 5'-ACGC GTNA-3'. This sequence is described as MCB *(Mlul* cell cycle box), since it represents a recognition site for *Mlul* enzyme.

Two protein factors, MBF factor and DSC1 (DNA synthesis) recognise MCB. A gene *cdc 10+* codes for a component of DSC1, which regulates *cdc22*$^{+}$ (gene for ribonucleotide reductase subunit), and possibly other genes of cell cycle. The *cdcl0*$^{+}$ gene product is believed to be a transcription factor like several other proteins involved in cell cycle. DNA damage checkpoint and Chkl. The DNA damage during cell division often leads to arrest of cell division either before DNA replication in Gl (this is called Gl checkpoint) or before mitosis in G2 (G2-M checkpoint). This response to DNA damage, leading to arrest of cell division is facilitated by regulation of Cdk-cyclin complexes, using checkpoint proteins. The checkpoints sense the DNA damage and transduce an inhibitory signal. Four genes (including *RAD9, RAD 17, RAD24, and MEC3)* will sense this DNA damage and are used for arrest of cell cycle at Gl and G2. The *cdcl3 rad9* double mutants fail to cause arrest suggesting that RAD9p should be sensor or transducer of DNA damage signal.

We know that in yeast, cdc2 protein remains inactive due to phosphorylation (at tyr's) and is activated by cdc25 (a phosphatase) through dephosphorylation. This phosphorylation also occurs on DNA damage and is maintained by the activity of protein kinase spWeel and the redundant spMikl (prefix sp means S. *pombe).* The model proposed for the DNA-damage checkpoint assumes, that DNA damage activates a protein spRad3, which in its active state brings about phosphorylation of Chkl. The phosphorylated form, Chkl-P functions as a kinase and brings about phosphorylation of cdc25 at Ser^{216}, which promotes binding of cdc25 to 14-3-3 (coded by *rad24* and *rad25),* leading to sequestration of cdc25. Consequently, cdc25 will not be available for activation of cdc2-P(tyr^{15}) so that the cell division will be arrested at G2-M transition (Fig.).

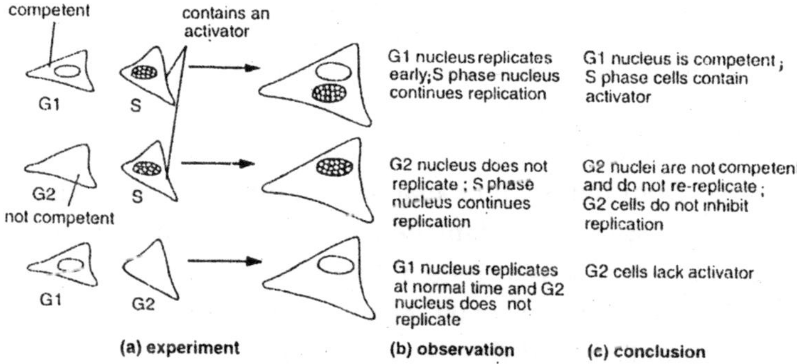

Results of cell fusion experiments involving cultured mammalian cells, showing factors that drive a G' nucleus directly into DNA synthesis and also showing that these factors, which present in S-phase cytoplasm and disappear in G2 phase.

Dependence of Centrosome Duplication on DNA Synthesis: When DNA synthesis is inhibited in the temperature sensitive yeast mutants, or when aphidicolin is added to mammalian cells, centrosome duplication is arrested. In yeast, due to a mutation *espl,* although DNA synthesis is blocked leading to inhibition of nuclear division, but centrosome duplication continues leading to accumulation of as many as eight centrosomes within the same cell. This proved the presence of a special gene *(espl+),* which prevents centrosome duplication in the absence of DNA synthesis.

Dependence of Mitosis on Spindle Function: It has been shown that a microtubular spindle is required for proper segregation of the chromosomes, so that an impaired spindle function leads to either an arrest of anaphase or to chromosome mis-segregation. This is suggested from the observation that whenever the spindle is disrupted with microtubular poisons, such as benomyl or nocodazole, progression through mitosis is blocked. In budding yeast *(S. cerevisiae)*, mutants have also been isolated which complete mitosis and cell division, even when spindle is not functioning properly.

What is the nature of this control, which prevents anaphase segregation of chromatids without proper spindle function? One possibility is that it operates by influencing inactivation of the $p34^{cdc2}$ kinase, normally required for successful completion of mitosis. If this inactivation of $p34^{cdc2}$ is not brought about, high $p34^{cdc2}$ activity will not allow the cell cycle to proceed from mitosis into anaphase, until this activity drops. Whenever spindle is damaged either by chemicals or by mutation, $p34^{cdc2}$ activity rises, although in *bub* and *mad* mutants, the $p34^{cdc2}$ activity can not be kept up, so that the cells gradually exit from mitosis and enter anaphase and then to interphase. The genes *BUB2, BUB3* and *MAD2* have been cloned and proteins encoded by them have been examined for their possible functions.

Spindle Assembly Checkpoint: A spindle assembly checkpoint is known to be present, which improves the fidelity of chromosome segregation by delaying anaphase until all chromosomes are correctly aligned on the mitotic spindle. It provides for a surveillance mechanism, which monitors the mitotic spindle connecting the chromosomes to the two pales with the help of their kinetochores. The checkpoint *firstly,* blocks the separation of two sister chromatids of a chromosome, until these two chromatids get attached to two opposite poles of the spindle and *secondly,* delays separation of chromatids in chromosomes already attached to spindle till such time that the kinetochores of all chromosomes are similarly attached. This type of control by checkpoint allows equal distribution of chromosomes to the two daughter cells.

With the discovery of the above checkpoint, it has recently been shown that kinetochores do not merely provide attachment sites for the spindle, but also control chromosome movement. It is believed that the kinetochores that are not yet attached

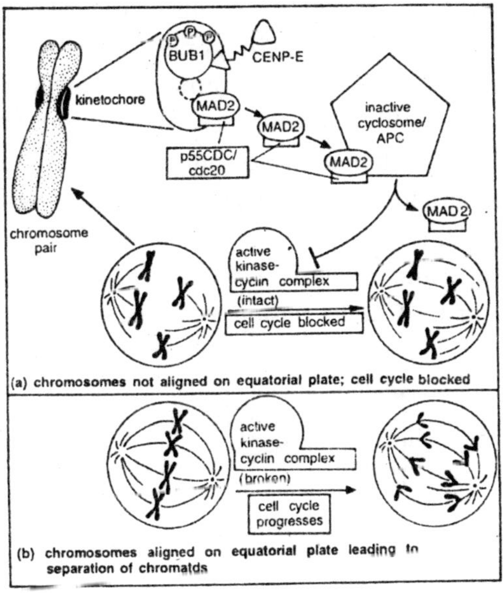

A model showing the operation of spindle assembly checkpoint.

to spindle fibres, release a signal (a 'wait' signal) in the form of a protein to keep a brake on cell division. When all the kinetochores are attached, the protein signal is somehow disabled thus releasing the brakes on mitosis. This was proved by the following two observations:

(i) If the unattached kinetochores are destroyed by a laser beam, the remaining chromosomes with attached kinetochores divided normally, thus proving that the unattached kinetochores do send a wait signal,

(ii) Some of the proteins at the kinetochores become dephos-phorylated, once the spindle fibres attach to the kinetochore.

In yeast, these proteins involved in sending the wait signal are encoded in two sets of genes, one including *BUB1, BUB2, BUB3 (bub* = budding uninhibited by benzimidazole) and the other including *MAD1, MAD2, MAD3 (mad* = mitotic arrest deficient). Corresponding mammalian genes recently identified included *MAD2* and *BUB1* in mice and *MAD2* in human. Mutants in *MAD* and *BUB* genes inactivate the spindle checkpoint. MAD2 protein remains concentrated at the kinetochore, until microtubules attachment is completed. Copies of this protein are also continuously migrating into the cytoplasm, broadcasting the wait signal throughout the cell. The signal is transmitted by association of MAD2 with p55CDC in mammals and of MAD2 with CDC20 in budding yeast (homolog of CDC20 in fission yeast is slp=sleepy).

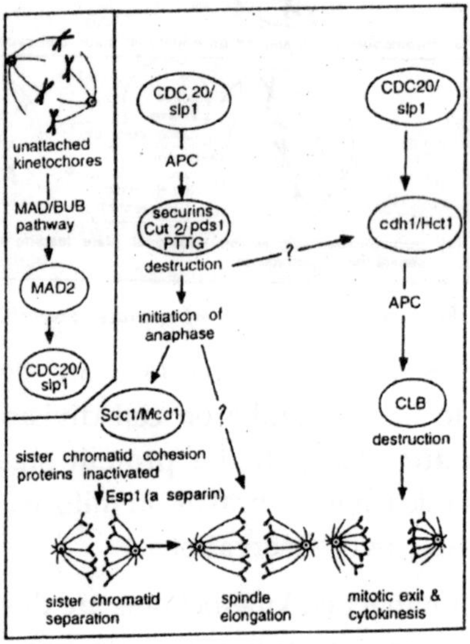

A model showing the role of CDC20 and Hctl in the degradation of CUT2/Pdsl and CLB2/Asel; these degradations are necessary for the success of anaphase.

When the interaction between these two proteins is disrupted, the spindle checkpoint is no longer functional. The two associated proteins (MAD2-p55CDC in mammals, MAD2-CDC20-in budding yeast and mad2-slpl in fission yeast) form a large protein complex called cyclosome or APC (anaphase promoting complex).

Another protein associated with APC is Hctl (cdhl in fission yeast). APC is kept in check by MAD2 and when active allows the cell to initiate anaphase (Fig.). APC helps initiation of anaphase by degradation of a group of proteins called securins, which include Cut2 in fission yeast, Pdsl in budding yeast and PTTG (an oncogene product) in vertebrates. Similarly Hctl controls degradation of B-type cyclins including CLB2 (Fig.). The degradation of securins triggers cleavage of a protein, called Sccl in budding yeast (Sccl, also called Mcdl, is a subunit of a multiprotein complex called cohesin). This cleavage of Sccl is facilitated by another protein Espl (called Cutl in *S. pombe*), a separin, which is actually responsible for the separation of sister chromatids.

It has also been proved for mammals, that BUB proteins (BUB1, BUB3) along with CENP-E protein (CENP-E helps in attachment of microtubule to the kinetochore and in the alignment of chromosomes at the equator) induce changes that ultimately shut down the transmission of 'wait' signal. These changes involve disabling of MAD2, which dissociates from p55CDC and loses its control on APC, so that APC is now activated and mitosis proceeds further. Active APC is believed to catalyze the breakdown of cyclins and other proteins which otherwise put the brakes on cell cycle. APC and Espl also remove cohesive proteins that keep the two chromatids of a chromosome together, thus facilitating separation of chromatids.

Dependence of Mitosis on Growth: The product of *weel* gene is not essential for mitosis (in *S. pombe*), but its presence delays mitosis. Deletion of *weel* or presence of its mutant allele gives cells smaller in size at mitosis and an increased dose of *weel* gives proportionately larger cells at mitosis. This suggests a genetic control of integration between growth and division.

Cell Division Controls in Multicellular Animals: Since many cells in adult multicellular animals stop dividing and only perform specialised function, they need positive signals (such as protein growth factors) to initiate cell division once again. This is in contrast to yeast, where a cell keeps on dividing, unless it receives a negative signal (such as mating type factor) to halt this proliferation.

The cell cycle genes in mammals have, however, been found to be similar to those described for yeast. For instance, Cdk gene *cdc2,* cyclin genes, and other genes like *cdc25* and *weel* are present in mammals also and if a mammalian gene is introduced into yeast lacking that gene, the yeast cells can be rescued.

However, the cell cycle control system in most multicellular organisms is more complex. As discussed earlier in this chapter, while in yeast, the same Cdk subunit is used at both G1/S and G_2/M transitions, different Cdks are used at these two stages in animal cells.

Growth Factors for Cell Proliferation and Cell Growth: We know that if yeast cells are deprived of nutrients, they stop dividing. Similarly, if mammalian cells are deprived of serum, they stop growing and become arrested between mitosis and S phase, in a quiescent state called GO (G zero). GO may also be achieved due to non-availability of appropriate growth factors. The serum contains growth factors needed only in very low concentration, each having a receptor (on cell surface) that responds to the growth hormone.

These growth factors can be proteins (atleast 50 such proteins are known) or other molecules, such as steroid hormones having intracellular receptors. Most of these growth factors stimulate cell proliferation as well as cell growth.

However, there are growth factors that stimulate only cell growth, such as nerve growth factor (NGF), which promotes growth of neurons. Some of these growth factors and their properties are given in Table. As can be noticed in this table some of these growth factors are such, which stimulate proliferation in" some cell types, and inhibit it in others.

Some Growth Factors Involved in Cell Proliferation and Cell Growth in Multicellular Organisms

Factor	*Representative action*
1. Plalelet derived growth factor (PDGF)	Stimulate proliferation of connective-tissue cells and some neuroglial cells.
2. Epidermal growth factor (EGF)	Stimulate proliferation of many cell types; act as inductive signal in embryonic development.
3. Insulin like growth factor I (IGF-I)	Promote cell survival, stimulate cell metabolism and collaborate with other growth factors.
4. Transforming regulate (TGF-p)	Influence response of cells to other growth factor β growth factors; differentiation of some cell types; act as inductive signals in embryonic development.
5. Fibroblast growth factor (FGF)	Stimulate proliferation in many cell types; inhibit differentiation of some stem cells; act as inductive signals in embryonic development.

Contd...

Factor	Representative action
6. Interleukin-2 (IL-2)	Stimulate proliferation of activated T lymphocytes of some neurons.
7. Nerve growth factor (NGF)	Promote survival and growth of nerve growth factors.
8. Erythropoietin	Promote proliferation, defferentiation and survival of red blood cell precursors.
9. Interleukin-3 (IL—3) precursors.	Stimulate proliferation and survival of various types of blood cell.

The ability of cells to enter GO in multicellular organisms accounts for enormous variability in the cell cycle of these organisms. For instance, in human body, neurons and skeletal muscle cells do not divide at all, liver cells divide only once every year, epithelial cells in the gut divide more than twice a day to renew the lining of the gut continuously. Cells in muticellular organisms also divide according to need. For instance, blood loss stimulates proliferation of blood cell precursors, acute liver damage provokes the surviving liver cells to proliferate, and the cells in the neighbourhood of a wound proliferate to repair the lesion.

The variation in the proliferation rates is due to the cells remaining in GO state for varying periods of time. GO state is often associated with depression in protein synthesis and is controlled by G1 checkpoint. This G1 checkpoint can be crossed only when adequate concentration of Cdk and Gl cyclin proteins are available. Protein growth factors in low concentration induce synthesis of Cdk and G1 cyclins, through a network of intracellular signaling cascades involving proto-oncogenies and tumour suppressor genes.

Cell Cycle and Cancer

During 1980's and 1990's, it became clear that derangements in the cell cycle machinery may actually be responsible for uncontrolled cell growth, characteristic of cancer. For instance, it has been shown that many oncogenes influence and stimulate cell division, even though indirectly. Tumour suppressor genes also operate through the molecular events during the cell cycle regulation so that a mutation for lack of function in any tumour suppressor gene may lead to cancer. For instance, the tumour suppressor gene *p53* is one of the commonest mutated (inactivated) gene in almost 50 per cent of all human cancers.

Intrinsic defects in the cell cycle machinery may also cause cancer. For instance, protein called cyclin D1 and several other proteins are the products of oncogenes. A group of cell cycle inhibitors also have the potential to be tumour suppressors, so that loss of these inhibitors may cause cancer. In view of the above, it is argued that once we understand the gene and gene products, which cause cancer, we may also design therapeutic strategies and new drugs for dealing with cancer. For instance, one may block the activation of cell cycle by inhibiting cyclin D1.

Cyclins (cyclin Dl, cyclin E, cyclin A) and Cdks in Cancer : Cyclin D1 is one of the eight or more cyclins known in mammals. If cyclin D1 is overproduced or produced at a wrong time, it would stimulate inappropriate cell divisions by keeping the corresponding Cdk (Cdk4, Cdk6) on, when it should be turned off. In 1991 the gene for cyclin D1 was found to be none else, but the oncogene *bell.* D cyclins are active at a critical time in the cell cycle, *i.e.*, G1 phase and decide whether the cell should enter DNA synthesis phase.

Once the DNA synthesis starts, the cell is committed to the rest of the cell cycle. Thus, amplification and over- expression of the gene for cyclin D1 were shown to cause a variety of cancers (breast, oesophagus, B cell lymphoma, etc.). Similarly cyclin E and cyclin A are usually active during the Gl phase of the cycle, but were found to be overexpressed in cancer cell lines. Some Cdks like Cdk4 have also been found to be amplified in some cancer cells.

Cell Cycle Inhibitors and Cancer: Loss of activity or function of some cell cycle inhibitors may also lead to cancer. These inhibitors include: (i) p53, which blocks the activity of Cdk2, and other Cdks, (ii) an inhibitor blocking specifically the Cdk4, and (iii) an inhibitor mediating TGF-p"s inhibitory effects.

Tumour Suppressors (p53 and Rb): Two important tumour suppressor genes include the following: (i) *p53* and (ii) *Rb* (retinoblastoma) gene. The suppressor gene *p53* has multifaceted activities but one of the important one involves its effector p21 (discovered only in 1993-94). This gene *p53* is known to control G1 phase, but recently its role in coordinating S and M phases of cell cycle has also been demonstrated.

The protein p53 has actually been dubbed as the 'guardian of the genome' or a 'watchman', so that conditions like DNA damage, hypoxia, oncogene activation and virus infection are sensed by p53, which in its turn either arrests the cell cycle through its effector p21 (a Cdk inhibitor) or else may cause the cell to kill itself (Fig.). If such an important is the role of p53, a mutation or defect in p53 may lead to uncontrolled cell division leading to cancer. Such mutant or defective cells will ignore DNA damage and other similar defects, which in a normal cell would warrant an arrest of cell division cycle. In view of this new information about the role of p53, antitumour therapies will be developed using this protein.

Aneuploidy and Cancer: A defect in spindle assembly checkpoint has also been found to cause aneuploidy associated with tumours (reported in 1998). One such defect was a mutation in *hBUBl* (h stands for human), a gene involved in spindle assembly checkpoint, so that the anaphase separation will be disrupted causing aneuploidy. It is possible that the missing chromosome(s) may carry tumour suppressor gene(s), whose absence may lead to uncontrolled cell division.

Meiotic Cell Division: During meiosis, two events, namely pairing of homologous chromosomes and recombination (exchange of chromosome segments) distinguish it from mitosis and therefore, have been the subject of intensive study. Sometimes a distinction has been made between presynaptic chromosome pairing and chromosome synapsis, the former implying alignment of homologous chromosomes, and the latter implying intimate association between them using SC (synaptonemal complex). Although the detailed molecular mechanisms underlying pairing, synapsis and recombination are still unknown, some clues have become available in recent years.

Recombination Precedes Synapsis in Yeast: Synapsis between homologous chromosomes, accompanies the formation of synaptonemal complex (SC) in early meiotic prophase I. This is generally believed to be a prerequisite for the meiotic recombination. However, recent studies in yeast have challenged this traditional view that chromosome synapsis is required for meiotic recombination. It has been shown in yeast that initiation of recombination precedes initiation of synapsis.

The evidence that synapsis follows recombination is available from the following observations: (i) the formation of double-strand breaks (DSBs) precedes SC formation; (ii) mutants that fail to create or process DSBs prevent the formation of SC; (iii) some mutants allow high level of recombination, but form no SC. If synapsis really follows recombination, single stranded DNA generated by a DSB carries out a homology search required for synapsis and SC formation.

In contrast to the above surprising situation in yeast, in fruitfly synapsis is independent of exchange of chromosome segments and can occur even in the absence of recombination. It is thus obvious that the molecular events in meiosis may differ in different organisms, particularly between organisms with small genomes and those with complex bigger genomes.

Drosophila Genes in Reduction Cell Division

In fruitfly, a set of genes have now been identified that regulate meiotic cell cycle and are necessary for segregation of chromosomes that do not undergo recombination. During meiosis, what holds the homologues together? SC can not perform this function, since it disappears in the diplotene, while the chromosomes remain together till metaphase I, and are believed to be held together due to chiasmata. But if chiasmata hold them together, how are the achiasmate chromosomes (*e.g.* chromosome IV in fruitfly) held together, and segregate faithfully? Mutations in genes *Axs, aid* and *mei-S51* affect the segregation of homologous non-exchange (achiasmate) chromosomes.

Two other genes needed for segregation are (i) *nod* (no distributive segregation and (ii) *ncd* (nonclaret disjunctional). Both encode microtubule motor proteins of kinesin family. Mutations in these two genes cause alterations in the pairing of chromosomes or spindle structure. A recently identified gene *Dub* (double or nothing) affects homologue segregation in meiosis I of males and females in *Drosophila*. *Dub* gene therefore may be responsible for chromosome pairing in both sexes.

Meiosis and Yeast Genes

In budding yeast, there are atleast three groups of genes regulating meiosis. These include *RAD, SPO* and *REC* genes. The genes of the *RAD52* epistasis group *(RAD50, RAD51, RAD52, RAD54, RAD55, RAD57, XRS2* and *MRE11)* are involved in both mitotic and meiotic recombination through DNA double-strand break (DSB) repair. Mutations in these genes lead to reduction in recombination. Three of these genes

(RAD51, RAD55, RAD57) and a related meiosis - specific yeast gene *(DMC1)* code for proteins that are similar to RecA, a protein important for prokaryotic recombination.

Rad51 is the most intensively studied of the RecA-like proteins in eukaryotes. Many proteins from the above Rad52 group in yeast physically interact with one another as shown through results of *in vitro* (biochemical) or *in vivo* systems using yeast two hybrid analysis. (In two hybrid system, a diploid strain is constructed, which carries two hybrid gene constructs, each having two components; one component in each gene construct encodes a protein and the other component each facilitates the study of physical interaction between the two proteins encoded in two hybrid gene constructs).

Following are some examples of such physical interactions: (i) Rad 51 interacts with Rad52, Rad54 and Rad53; (ii) Rad52 interacts with Rad51; (iii) Rad55 interacts with Rad57; (iv) Mrell *'(BC-27)* interacts with Rad50 and Xrs2. These observations suggest that proteins of Rad52 group function together with other proteins as multi-protein complexes in DNA repair and recombination. Other studies also revealed that Rad51 has a role in meiotic recombination in higher eukaryotes.

Several *SPO* (sporulation) genes have also been identified in budding yeast. For instance *SPO13* gene temporarily blocks entry into meiosis to allow time for assembly of the reductional segregation apparatus. Mutants for such *SPO* genes *(spoil, spol3)* cause early reduction division. There is another set of genes *(REC102, REC104, REC114* and *ME 114)* which coordinate recombination with reduction division. *REC102, REC104* and *REC114* are early exchange genes and mutations in these genes cause early reduction division.

In fission yeast (*S. pombe)* also there are about 40 *rec* genes for recombination. Mutations in these genes lead to 10 to 1000 fold reduction in recombination (based on the study of intragenic recombination at *ade6* locus). Many of these genes have been cloned and sequenced and some of them show homology with genes of budding yeast (*e.g.* Rec 12 amino acid sequence shares identity with Spoil of budding yeast).

Importance of MPF during Reduction Cell Division: Frog oocyte and egg have been widely used for the study of shift from mitotic cell division to meiotic cell division. The major events from immature oocyte (primary oocyte) to the early mitotic cell divisions in the zygote are shown in Figure

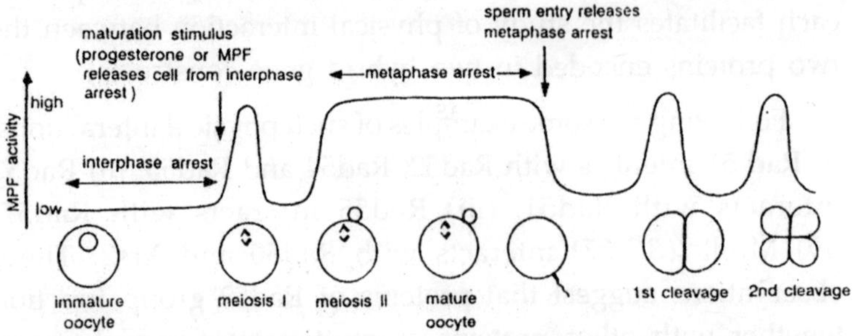

Early frog life cycle: the appearance of frog egg and oocyte and the level of MPF activity are shown during meiosis, fertilization and early development of zygote. Points of cell cycle arrest and the stimuli that release these arrests are also indicated.

The cell cycle remains arrested at G2 in interphase before meiotic division and secretion of progesterone (extracellular) by the follicle cells induces the oocyte to proceed rapidly through meiosis I and prophase of meiosis II, before arresting it at metaphase of meiosis II.

The immature eggs were also shown to produce MPF described earlier for mitotic cell division, so that MPF activity (discovered initially in egg for meiosis) is needed for mitosis as well as meiosis, and is associated with metaphase state. It was also shown that the rise in MPF activity was dependent on protein synthesis, although it was not clear whether the newly synthesized component was MPF itself or its activity.

Biochemistry of Chromosome Pairing in Meiosis: The structure and function of synaptonemal complex and recombination nodules associated with chromosome pairing and crossing over respectively. These structures are morphological manifestations of the mechanism that may be controlling these phenomena. However, the study of biochemistry associated with these morphological structures may be more difficult to study.

Chromosome pairing, however, is the major distinction between mitosis and meiosis and one would like to know the mechanism responsible for making this distinction. Despite concerted efforts in this direction very little is known about the biochemical basis of chromosome pairing. Further, although we know many mutations (asynapsis, desynapsis, diploidising genes, etc.) which regulate chromosome pairing, but none of these genes could be isolated or cloned, nor could we isolate the product of any of these genes.

In *Drosophila*, during mid 1990's evidence became available suggesting that atleast some of the chromosome pairing is initiated or maintained by the heterochromatin (found at the centromere and terminal regions of chromosomes), consisting mainly of non-coding repetitive sequences. In several chromosomes (particularly the tiny chromosome IV), achiasmate disjunction involving pairing followed by segregation without associated recombination has been demonstrated.

The early nodules may be involved in searching for DNA homology before synaptic initiation. Two components of these nodules are RAD51 and DMC1 proteins, which are homologous to RecA of prokaryotes involved in pairing and exchange of DNA strands. DMC1 in yeast and LIM15 of lily colocalise with RAD51. Both RAD51 and DMC1 proteins are believed to be important for chromosome pairing.

During the last two decades, studies have also been conducted on DNA synthesis during the different phases of meiotic cell cycle in lily *(Lilium)*. It was shown that a group of single or low copy number DNA sequences (3×10^7 bp) that constitute 0.1 to 0.2 per cent of the genome do not replicate during the premeiotic S-phase. This small fraction of DNA replicates instead at zygotene in coordination with chromosome pairing. This is called zyg DNA (or zygotene DNA) and occurs in segments averaging about 4-5 kb (range 2.5-10 kb) in length and is broadly distributed among all the chromosomes.

Zyg DNA replication occurs after the meiotic cells have entered prophase, but is not completed at zygotene or soon after. Single strand gaps remain at the ends of the otherwise replicated zyg DNA segments until sometime after pachytene, when the synaptonemal complex begins to disassemble. Zyg DNA is transcribed into poly $(A)^+$ RNA at a time, when the chromosomes initiate pairing process. This 'zyg RNA' has not been detected in nonmeiotic tissues.

Even within the meiocytes, zyg RNA is not detectable prior to leptotene or beyond mid-pachytene. In mouse spermatocytes also, the profile of zyg RNA formation and disappearance is very similar to that of zyg RNA in lily meiocytes. Further, no zyg RNA has been detected in mouse somatic tissues. In contrast to zyg DNA, there is another group of DNA sequences called pachytene DNA, which undergoes a programmed repair replication, once pairing is complete.

Dynamics of Chromosome Movements During Cell Division

Events Involving Chromosome Movement: Chromosomes are involved in a series of directed movements during both mitosis and meiosis. During mitosis, where chromosome movements have been studied in some detail, following events have been observed, which are shown in Figure. In prometaphase, chromosomes move (.05 to 1.0 mm sec^{-1}) and attach to spindle microtubules both terminally and laterally, and atleast in some cases, can be seen together at the spindle poles. (Microtubules are unbranched tube like structures, present in the cell, and mainly consist of a protein called tubulin; they are involved in the structure of cilia, flagelle and spindle and help in movements of cilia, flagella and chromosomes.

Microtubules provide the framework for the mitotic spindle, and are oriented with their so called minus (-) ends at the spindle poles and their plus (+) ends overlapping in the centre of the spindle. As prometaphase progresses, the speed of chromosomes slows down (.01 to .05 μ m sec^{-1}). Subsequently, after a slow bidirectional shuffle, the chromosomes migrate towards the mid-zone of the spindle through a process called congression and form the metaphase plate.

After this, in a coordinated manner, the chromosomes split and proceed towards the spindle poles with slow and uniform motion. This stage is anaphase, which has two parts, anaphase A and anaphase B. Anaphase A (earlier part of anaphase) involves specific shortening of microtubules associated with kinetochore (discontinuous microtubules), while anaphase B (later part) involves elongation of the entire spindle (continuous microtubules).

Kinetochore and Spindle in Chromosome Movement: Kinetochore, which is coincident with the centromere and is a trilaminar plate situated at the primary constriction (or centromere) of the chromosome, plays an important role in chromosome movements. It is through these specialised structures called kinetochores, that the chromosomes get attached to microtubules (Fig.) and help in their movement during anaphase. Recent studies have also shown that kinetochores are sites for generation of force required for chromosome movement.

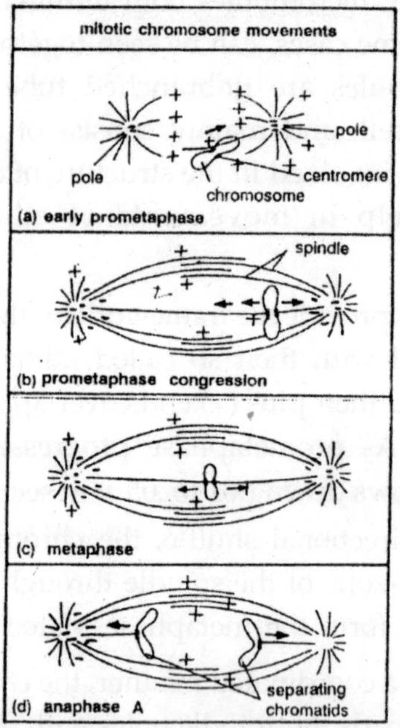

Events of chromosome movements during mitosis. In prometaphase, the chromatid pair is first drawn to the spindle pole, then migrates towards the centre of the spindle. At the onset of anaphase, the chromatids separate and migrate slowly towards the spindle poles.

Following generalisations (based on experiments) have been made regarding kinetochore, spindle apparatus, centrosome and interactions between them: (i) At the time of spindle formation, there is an increase in phosphorylation of several proteins, (ii) Kinetochore microtubules (MTs) can both add (polymerisation) and lose (depolymerisation) subunits at or near the kinetochores; similarly, subunits addition (polymerisation) at the centrosome-distal ends of NiTs leads to elongation of continuous fibres, (iii) Kinetochores are capable of both binding to and sliding on the microtubules. (iv) During formation of spindle at prometaphase, a chromosome is under tension from both ends of the spindle, so that a centrosome directed force is acting at each kinetochore. (v) Kinetochore-spindle fibre interactions are unstable, until there is an opposing force which may resist chromosome movement; this may stabilise chromosome attachment, the stability being dependent on proper orientation of chromosome with respect to spindle. Thus improper chromosome orientations will not survive, (vi) A single centrosome pulls on a kinetochore and pushes off the rest of the chromosome. This duality of forces may be significant for prometaphase motion of chromosomes to metaphase plate, (vii) Once the spindle is established at metaphase, the centrosome becomes dispensable, (viii) Kinetochore- centrosome attractions result in chromosome movement, so that when two chromatids separate, they move automatically towards the poles, due to disassembly (depolymerisation) of microtubules attached to kinetochores. (ix) The force acting on anaphase chromosomes is 7 × 10 dynes, (x) The discontinuous spindle fibres carrying the kinetochores contract and pull the chromosomes towards the poles, while the continuous fibres elongate and hold the poles apart.

Basic Questions about Kinetochore Function: Two basic questions about the function of kinetochore, which are being actively pursued are: (i) how do microtubules get attached to kinetochores? and (ii) what are the structural requirements for the generation of the force required for chromosome movement? Both these questions have been partly answered through experiments conducted during 1990's

Mechanism of Kinetochore-microtubule Attachment: Following two hypotheses were earlier available for kinetochore-microtubule attachment: (i) According to first hypothesis, the microtubules are nucleated at the centrosome and later captured by the kinetochores. (ii) According to second hypothesis the microtubules are nucleated at the kinetochores, and only later interact with the spindle pole. Recently, support for the first hypothesis was provided by video contrast optical microscopy. It was possible to image individual microtubules, as they grow out from mitotic poles and first come in contact with kinetochores. Contact is established as a microtubule grows out towards the periphery of the spindle, brushing past the side of a kinetochore.

Dynamic instability causes continuous growth and shrinkage of microtubules, allowing them to probe through the cytoplasm and thus increasing the probability of finding kinetochores. The kinetochore latches into the microtubule lattice and the chromosome is jerked polewards (Fig.). A motor protein dynein, which is now known to be a part of kinetochore, may be involved in this movement. However, the possibility that the chromosomes are pulled polewards by microtubule depolymerisation, can not be ruled out.

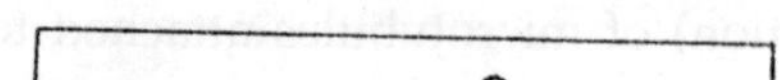
microtubule shrinks back
kinetochore
microtubule growing out
(a) several microtubules grow out or shrink back to spindle pole
vesicle
(b) a microtubule interacts laterally with kinetochore
chromosome
vesicle
chromosome moving polewards
Shrink
(c) a vesicle makes contact with same microtubule

The process of microtubule attachment to the kinetochore. (a) Several microtubules grow out from, and shrink back towards, the spindle pole during prometaphase. (b) One microtubule makes a lateral contact with a kinetochore; the kinetochore attaches to it and starts moving polewards, (c) A vesicle makes a lateral contact with the same microtubule and also moves polewards.

Mechanism of anaphase chromosome movement. According to an earlier view, the kinetochore is a passive structure, which remains attached to microtubule ends, while these microtubules are shortened. The shortening of microtubules is achieved by disassembly or depolymerisation. In this hypothesis, energy released (from GTP hydrolysis) during the microtubule assembly and disassembly is sufficient to drive chromosome movement during anaphase A, and any role of motor molecules was ruled out.

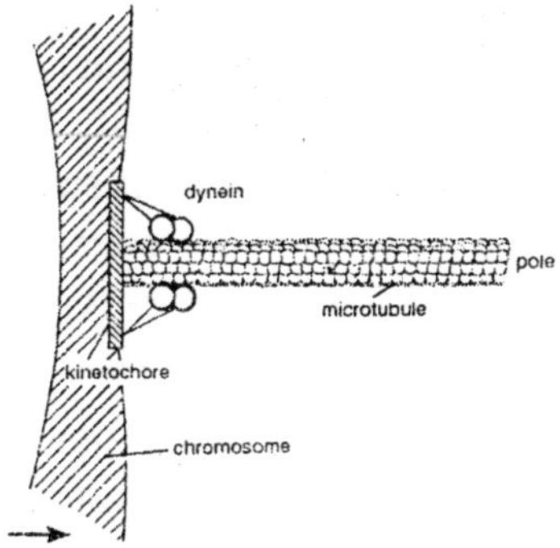

Possible arrangement of dynein in the kinetochore; two headed dynein molecules are shown tugging on the end of a microtubule, whose disassembly could govern rate of movement.

However, recently kinetochore has been shown to be a dynamic structure, which may contain two force producing ATPases in the form of proteins like kinesin and cytoplasmic dynein (Fig.). The forces generated by these two motor proteins are opposite in direction, one of them directed towards the pole and the other away from it. In this hypothesis, energy for the force is released during hydrolysis of ATP involved in phosphorylation of motor proteins.

The presence of cytoplasmic dynein and its association with kinetochore was recently demonstrated by immunofluorescence microscopy, but no such cytological evidence for the presence of kinesin could be available (although the presence of a kinesin like motor protein was inferred from other observations). Dramatic evidence for rapid chromosome movement along microtubules *in vivo* has also been presented, which suggests a role of motor molecules in chromosome movement during anaphase A. One of the obvious candidates for such a motor molecule is cytoplasmic dynein, which produces force in the appropriate direction to make the chromosomes move towards the spindle poles. However, the rates of chromosome movement during metaphase and anaphase (1-3 μm min^{-1} or .01–.05 μm sec^{-1}) are much slower than those expected from dynein.

In Vitro Association and Relative Movement of Microtubules and Kinetochores: Recently the forces involved in chromosome movements have been studied using *in vitro* techniques involving association of isolated chromosomes and microtubules. The association and chromosome movement were recorded using video microscopy.

Since, it is difficult to examine the movement of relatively large chromosomes along very thin microtubules, in this recent *in vitro* study the movement of microtubules against the chromosomes, adsorbed on a slide, was examined. In order to detect the movement of microtubules and its direction, the microtubules were assembled from a mixture of fluorescently labelled and unlabelled tubulin subunits, so that the minus (-) or pole ends and the plus (+) ends of microtubules could be distinguished by the intensity of fluorescence.

Association in Presence of ATP: It was shown that microtubules become associated with kinetochores and in presence of ATP (to add phosphate group) travel towards the minus end (or in poleward direction). The rate of movement was 0.46 μm sec^{-1} (28 μm min^{-1}), similar to that in early prometaphase, but much greater than the known rate of chromosome movement during anaphase.

This was explained on the basis of the assumption that chromosomes were perhaps isolated from cells arrested at prometaphase. The movement can be attributed to cytoplasmic dynein, which has already been implicated in early prometaphase movement. Dynein may be involved in poleward movement in early prometaphase as well as during anaphase.

Another protein (kinesin) may be involved in reverse movement towards centre during congression.

Association after Pertreatment with ATP-v-S: When the chromosomes and microtubules were pretreated with ATP-v-S (with thiophosphate group) before adding ATP, the movement was much slower (.048 μ m/sec^{-1}). and in opposite direction, *i.e.,* towards the centre.

ATP-v-S will add a thiophosphate group preferentially to one motor protein, which can not be removed by a phosphatase so that the protein is modified irreversibly, thus turning off the minus-end directed motors and turning on the plus-end directed motors. Using an antibody (anti-thiophosphate), this thiophosphate group could be located in the kinetochore, suggesting that phosphorylation of a component protein of kinetochore actually leads to reversal of the direction of chromosome movement. It is suggested that both a kinase (it could be *cdc-2* kinase) and a phosphatase may be associated with the kinetochore (kinase adds phosphate group and phosphatase removes it). Further, there may be two motor proteins (dynein and kinesin) involved in the development of forces in opposite directions.

Role of Phosphorylation in Motor Activity: Using *in virto* studies, it could be shown that there are two types of motor proteins at the kinetochores, one developing minus-end directed force and the other developing a plus-end directed force. ATP analogues (*e.g.* ATP-v-S) were used which are known to be used differently by known motor proteins, dynein and kinesin, both ATPases. The minus-end motor gives a response similar to that given by dynein, which has now been shown to be located at kinetochore. But plus-end motor protein seems to be different from kinesin (GTP is used by kinesin, but not by plus-end motor protein; also kinesin makes microtubules move much faster), which unlike dynein could not be located in kinetochore. Thus it may be a new protein.

It has also been shown that differential phosphorylation and dephosphorylation of two ATPases (motor proteins) in kinetochores are responsible for chromosome movements during cell division. The phosphorylation is facilitated by a kinase enzyme and dephosphorylation is facilitated by a phosphatase enzyme, and a delicate balance between kinase and phosphatase is maintained. Although it is not known how phosphorylation controls direction of motor movement, but a parallelism has been drawn with similar control system in melanophores, where pigment movement is effected by two motors, whose relative activities are controlled by phosphorylation. Besides phosphorylation and dephosphorylation, microtubules grow and shrink (due to polymerisation and depolymerisation) at the kinetochore. This suggests that motor activity and microtubule dynamics are coordinated in a delicate manner regulating chromosome movement, away from and towards the spindle pole during cell division.

Reversible phosphorylation within a cell is such an important phenomenon in cellular regulatory mechanisms, that the 1992 Nobel Prize for medicine was awarded to two U.S. bio-chemists (Edmond Fischer and Edwin Krebs) for their researches in this area.

Role of Degradation of Proteins (Proteolysis) in Cell Cycle: Initially, during 1980's, research in cell division cycle suggested that the cell cycle is regulated mainly by the timely synthesis of several regulatory proteins like Cdks, cyclins, Cdk inhibitors, and other kinases (*e.g.* Caks), phosphatases and some unknown non-cyclin proteins. However, later during mid-1990s, there was a major shift in emphasis towards the study of timely destruction of key proteins (proteolysis) during the progress of cell cycle. This proteolysis was found to play a major role in regulating the events in cell cycle. The proteolysis was also found to be facilitated by the protein ubiquitin which forms a 26S proteasome with the target proteins to be destroyed. A biochemical machinery has also been found to exist, which controls these events of proteolysis. Proteolysis actually involves degradation of the following proteins at three checkpoints: (i) cyclins ; (ii) inhibitors of the activity of CDKs and that of its components, (iii) a putative protein that is a chromosome tether and holds chromatids together; it needs to be degraded before chromatids separate.

It has also been shown recently that proteolysis does not merely regulate CDK activity for the progression of cell cycle, but may also independently and directly control a step in cell cycle such as chromosome segregation at anaphase. It has been shown that mutants lacking the ability to bring about the desired proteolysis at specific checkpoints in the cell cycle, exhibit uncontrolled cell growth and cancer. For instance, once a Cdk-cyclin complex (CDK) has done its job, cyclin undergoes proteolysis. In a mutant where cyclin can not undergo proteolysis (as also observed due to removal of nine amino acids from one end), the cells are stuck in mitosis. These nine

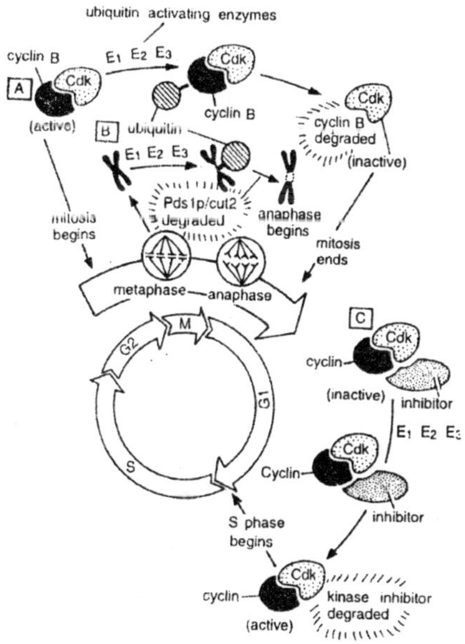

Ubiquitination of cell cycle proteins with the help of three enzymes, as a prerequisite for degradation.

amino acid residues at one end of a cyclin were later shown to be necessary for attachment of cyclin to ubiquitin, which facilitates degradation.

In addition to cyclins, several proteins acting as inhibitors of the activity of Cdks also need to be degraded before Cdk can become active to perform its function. Some non-cyclin proteins that hold chromatids together during G2 and metaphase also need to be degraded before anaphase segregation is brought about. One such inhibitory protein is p40 (Sicl) in yeast which needs to be degraded with the help of ubiquitin, before CDK is activated to initiate DNA synthesis. Another mammalian CDK inhibitor is p27 which undergoes degradation with the help of ubiquitin.

Factors Determining which Proteins to be Degraded and when: Proteolysis is so important for the progress of cell cycle, that one would like to study the factors which will not only identify the proteins that need to be subjected to proteolysis,

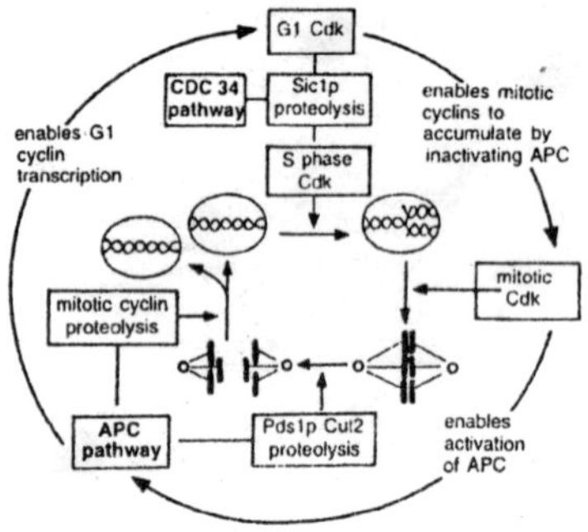

C34 pathway and APC
of cell cycle through

Two proteolytic pathways (CDC34 pathway and APC pathway), which regulate progression of cell cycle through interaction with CDKs.

but will also determine the time for such proteolysis. Three enzymes called El, E2 and E3 (letter E was used, because these were first defined as eluates from ubiquitin affinity column) are known to be involved in the attachment of ubiquitin to the protein that needs to be degraded (Fig.). While E2 remains active throughout the cell cycle, E3 has a temporal control (temporal control means it will be active at a specific time).

Following two distinct proteolytic pathways interacting with CDKs are now known for successful completion of cell cycle (Fig.) (i) The first pathway (called CDC34 pathway) promotes progression of G1 to S phase and utilises E2 called CDC34 in budding yeast (several different E2s are known).

The gene *CDC34* encodes a ubiquitin conjugating enzyme that helps ubiquitination leading to the destruction of multiple proteins, which include not only Gl cyclins, CLN2 and CLN3 (three cyclins namely CLN1, CLN2 and CLN3 drive cells through G1 by activating CDC28 in budding yeast), but also other proteins not directly related to cell cycle control. CDC34 is also involved in proteolysis of a CDK inhibitor namely Sicl in yeast and p27 in human cells, whose presence blocks transition from G1 to S phase. Three other genes involved in G1-S transition include *CDC4, CDC5* and *SKP1*. Their function at the molecular level will be known in future.

It has, however, been shown that phosphorylation of cyclins, CLN2 and CLN3 and also that of CDK inhibitor Sicl is necessary for CDC34-dependent ubiquitination. (ii) The second pathway (called APC pathway) involves metaphase-anaphase transition. The degradation of cyclin B (mitotic cyclins) is required for the exit form telophase, but the degradation of other substrates is needed for anaphase progression. The mitotic cyclins contain a conserved 9-amino acid motif called D Box (destruction box), which is necessary for ubiquitination and subsequent degradation. In contrast to CDC34 pathway, where phosphorylation of substrate is necessary for degradation, no phosphorylation of cylcin B is required for its degradation. The ubiquitination of cyclin B does utilise two E2 enzymes (UBC4 and UBCx or E2-C). A large E3 complex known as cyclosome or the anaphase-promoting complex (APC) is also needed for proteolysis that is essential for anaphase progression in many organisms. It has been shown now that non-degradable forms of mitotic cyclins arrest the cell cycle in telophase rather than metaphase both in *Xenopus* and budding yeast.

Therefore, sister chromatid segregation is not triggered by MPF inactivation, but by the degradation of some non-cyclin proteins that inhibit anaphase separation of chromatids and thus are believed to be the putative chromosome tether proteins. This degradation is brought about by APC-mediated proteolysis. Two such non-cyclin proteins include Cut2 in fission yeast and Pdsl in budding yeast.

While phosphorylation of proteins (Cdks, cyclins) during cell cycle is reversible, proteolysis is irreversible and thus performs two functions:

(i) it provides direction to the critical steps in cell cycle and

(ii) it regulates timing of the cell cycle transitions.

Thus CDK activity and proteolysis are interdependent and ensure that events in the cell cycle occur in proper order.

7

Adhesive Character

Cell Adhesion

The cells in tissues are assembled together and remain in contact with the help of extracellular matrix (ECM). These tissues in vertebrates include nerve, blood, lymphoid, epithelial and connective tissues. Among these tissues, at one extreme is the connective tissue in which cells are sparsely distributed and ECM is abundant bearing most of the mechanical stress. On the other extreme is the epithelial tissue, where cells are tightly bound together into sheets called epithelia and ECM is scanty consisting of a thin basal lamina, so that cells themselves bear most of the stress with the help of cytoskeleton. The cells in all these tissues are held together by cell-cell adhesion, which may or may not be associated with the formation of structures called 'cell junctions'.

In early stages of development, only cell-cell adhesions are displayed and no cell junctions are observed under the microscope, but in mature adult structures, cell junctions can be observed under the electron microscope. While the cell-cell adhesions have been studied through functional and biochemical tests, particularly in embryonic tissues during development, the cell junctions have been studied by electron microscopy, particularly in the mature adult structures. In recent years, a unified picture of these cell adhesions and cell junctions has also emerged due to an understanding of their molecular basis. In this chapter, we first discuss the functional and biochemical aspects of cell-cell adhesion and then describe the structure and function of different types of cell junctions.

Differential Cell Relationship

Cell sorting is a phenomenon, which allows different types of cells to segregate and form specific regions of the developing embryo. Therefore, in recent years, a study of cell sorting helped in understanding the mechanism involved in the normal development of the embryo. Although the cell surface looks much the same in all cells, it actually differs in different cell types and facilitates cell sorting through cell-cell interactions. A definite evidence suggesting the presence of the phenomenon of 'cell sorting' was actually provided by Townes and Holtfreter in the year 1955.

They demonstrated that the dissociated cells of vertebrate embryonic organs can reaggregate and sort out to reconstruct semblances (structures looking alike) of the original structure. The amphibian tissues do become dissociated into single cells when placed in alkaline solution. Utilising this feature, Townes and Holtfreter prepared single cell suspensions from each of the three germ layers (ectoderm, mesoderm, endoderm) soon after the neural tube had formed in amphibian embryos. It could be shown that when cells of different kinds were mixed, cells of same type aggregated together through the phenomenon of cell adhesion.

The result of these experiments led to the following conclusions: (i) The reaggregated cells become spatially segregated in the reconstructed structures. (ii) The reaggregated cells reflected the embryonic positions; for instance, when ectodermal and mesodermal cells are mixed, they sort out and ectodermal cells are found at periphery, while mesodermal cells are found inside, so that epiderm envelopes the mesoderm (Fig.); the mesoderm also migrates centrally with respect to endoderm or gut (Fig.); similarly, when cells from three layers are mixed, the endoderm separates from ectoderm and mesoderm and is then enveloped by them; the neural plate cells also migrate to their corresponding position.

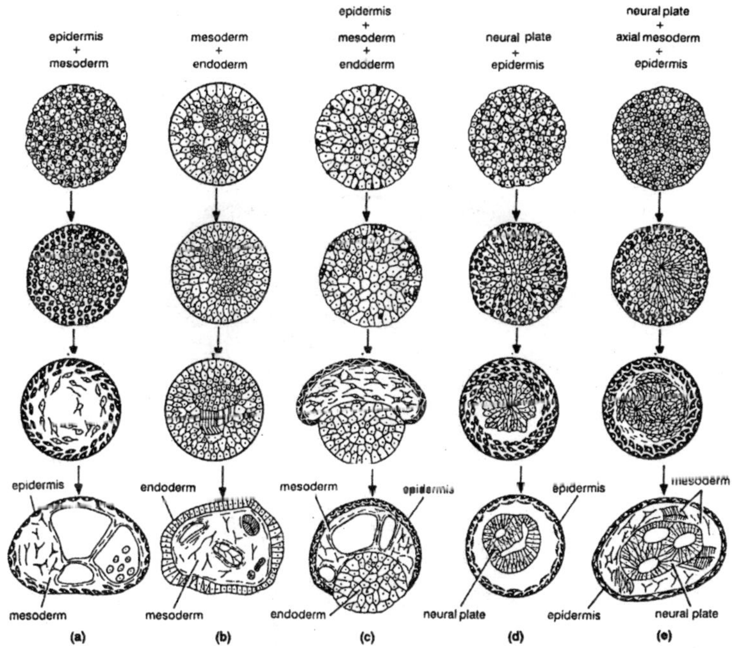

Sorting out of the aggregates of embryonic cells and reoganisation of their spatial relationships (redrawn from Gilbert, 1994).

These results were interpreted in terms of relative positive affinity of the inner surface of ectoderm for mesoderm, and its negative affinity for endoderm; mesoderm in its turn had positive affinity both for ectoderm and endoderm. (iii) The selective affinities of cells change during development; for instance, in blastula, all cells seem to have same affinity for each other but have high affinity for the extracellular matrix or ECM (hyaline layer) covering of the embryo and low affinity for the proteins inside the blastocoel. At the onset of gastrulation, a specific group of cells at the vegetal end of the blastula lose their affinity for neighbouring cells and for external extracellular matrix, but acquire affinity for protein fibrils inside the blastocoel.

Consequently, the cells release their contacts with adjoining cells and migrate inside the blastocoel, where they form the skeleton (Fig.). These changes in affinities are accompanied with changes in adhesion properties and are extremely important during morphogenesis.

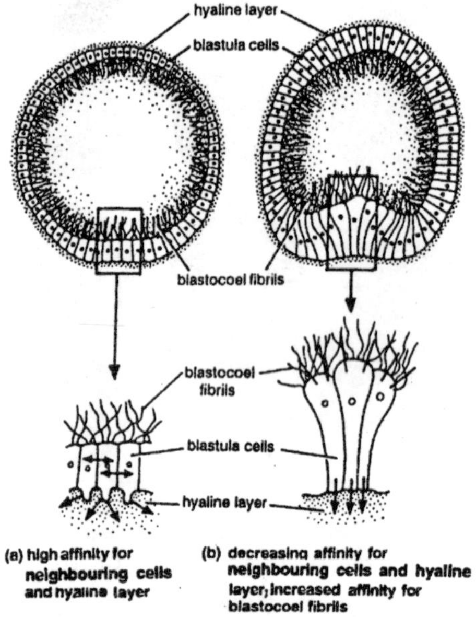

Changes in cell adhesion properties of skeletal precursor cells with development (redrawn from Gilbert, 1994).

Cell Connected Molecules

Differentiation and morphogenesis during development of multicellular organisms involve a variety of interactions among different cells or between cells and its external environment. One of these interactions involves the phenomenon of selective cell recognition and cell adhesion, which may include adhesion among adjoining cells forming tissues, or between cells and the substratum leading to attachment of the cell.

Cell adhesion is mediated by cell adhesion molecules (CAMs), substratum adhesion molecules and cell junction molecules (Fig.). These molecules (excluding cell junctions) include the following four major families of receptors: (i) cadherins, whose adhesion properties are dependent on Ca^{++} ions; (ii) members of Ig superfamily (they are Ca^{++} independent) including N-CAM (neural cell-cell adhesion molecules) and ICAM-1 (intercellular adhesion molecules, whose cell binding domains resemble those of immunoglobulin molecules); (iii) selectins and (iv) integrins. The first three of these molecules mediate cell-cell adhesion, while integrins mediate cell-substratum adhesion.

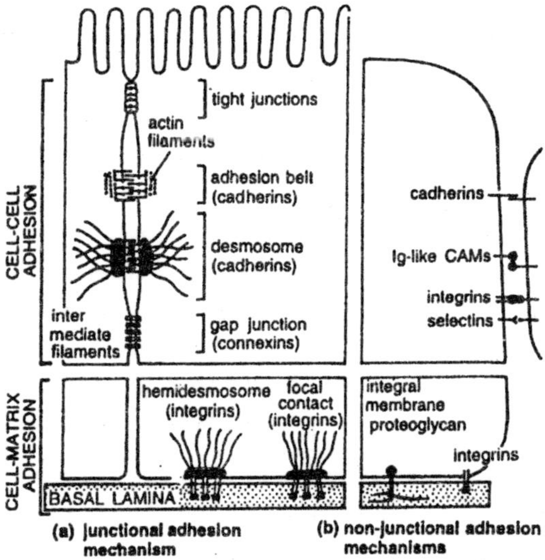

Junctional and non-junctional adhesive mechanisms used by animal cells (redrawn from Alberts et. al., Molecular Biology of the Cell, 1994).

Cadherins (Ca^{++} Dependent Cell-cell Adhesion): Cadherins are calcium-dependent glycoproteins, which are crucial to the spatial segregation of cells leading to the organisation of animal form. In mammalian embryos, following three classical cadherins are found (although 12 different types are known): (i) E-cadherins (epithelial cadherins, also called uvomorulins or L-CAM); (ii) P-cadherins (placental cadherins) and (iii) N-cadherins (neural cadherins, also called A-CAM). It has been shown that cells with a particular type of cadherins adhere preferentially to other cells' expressing the same cadherins. This is called homophilic binding (Fig.). Each cadherin has three major regions - an NH_2-terminal extracellular recognition domain of 113- amino acids (containing four major repeats) outside the cell, a transmembrane domain spanning the membrane and cytoplasmic domain within the cell. The extracellular domain differs among cadherins and help in cell-sorting or cell recognition and is also responsible for Ca^{++} binding. The cytoplasmic domain mediates interaction with atleast three cytosolic proteins called α -, β - and γ -catenins. Although extracellular domain helps in cell recognition, but no cadherin mediated cell adhesion is observed in cells lacking either the cytoplasmic domain of cadherin or one of the three cytosolic proteins, the α -, β - and γ - catenins (Figures). It is postulated that in the presence of Ca^{++}, the carboxy terminal cytoplasmic domain of a cadherin is connected to actin microfilaments of the cytoskeleton through the catenins. The clustering of cadherins, catenins and actins in this manner leads to the formation of a belt-like region called adherens-junction or zonulae adherens, which is responsible for cell- cell adhesion. It has also been shown that the integrity of these junctions is regulated by protein-tyrosine phosphorylation.

Another example of cell-cell adhesion is represented by 'desmosomes' (also called 'maculla adherens'), which are spot-like sites of intercellular contact. In this case, the cell adhesion is mediated by three transmembrane Ca^{++} dependent proteins (desmoglein I, desmocollin I and desmocollin II), each with four external extracellular domains identical to those found in classical cadherins. However, the cytoplasmic domains differ and are linked to intermediate filaments (not to actins as found in classical cadherins), through a cytoplasmic structure called the desmosomal plaque (Fig.). Cadherins are extremely important in establishment and maintenance of cell-cell interactions and their deficiency may lead to malignancy of cells or to other life threatening diseases like pemphigus vulgaris, in which epidermal cells lose adhesion, blister and fall off.

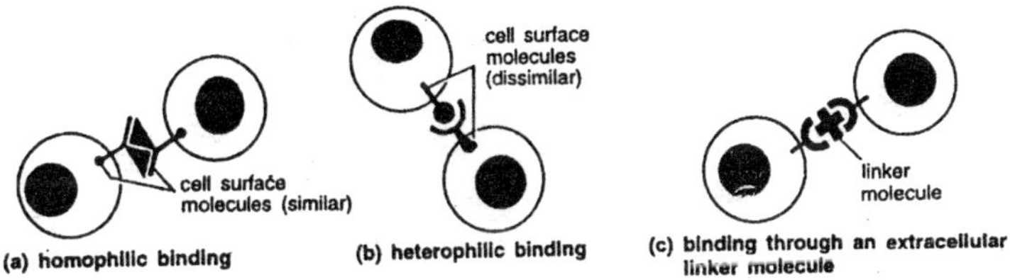

Three mechanisms by which cell surface molecules can mediate cell-cell adhesion (redrawn from Alberts et. al., Molecular Biology of the Cell, 1994).

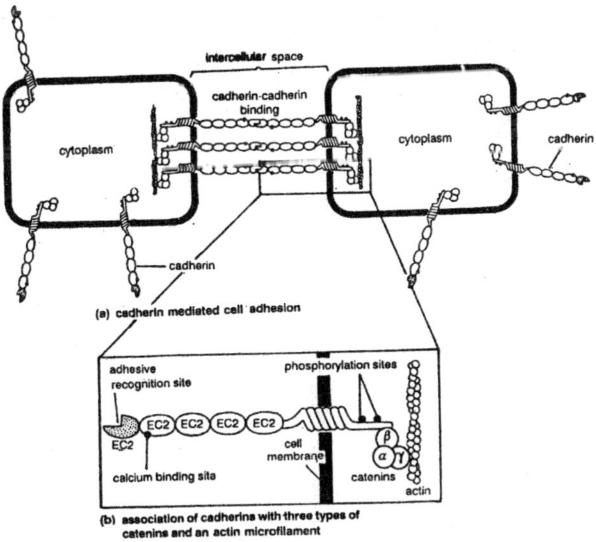

Cadherin mediated cell adhesion involving association of cadherins with three types of catenins and an actin microfilament (redrawn from Gilbert, 1994).

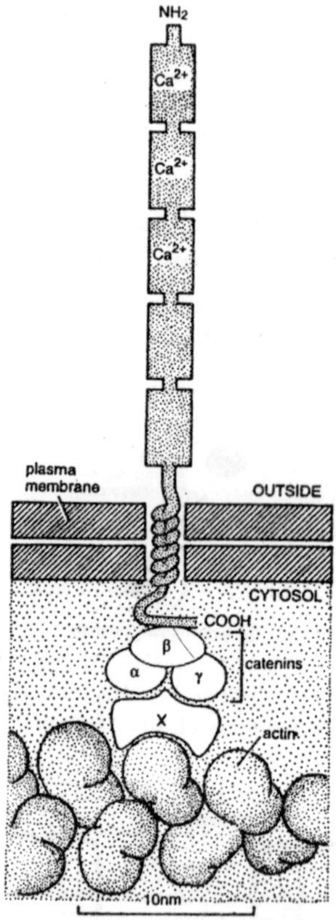

Structure of a cadherin molecule with five extracellular domains, three of them having calcium binding sites, the farthest of which mediates cell-cell adhesion (redrawn from Alberts et. al., Molecular Biology of the Cell, 1994).

Immunoglobulin Superfamily CAMs (Ca^{++} Independent Cell-cell Adhesion): As the word 'superfamily' implies, these immunoglobulin related cell adhesion molecules (CAMs) are large and varied. They are the most populous and represent a functionally diverse family of molecules present on the cell surface. (The designation 'superfamily' is used because immunoglobulins themselves constitute a family, and these immunoglobulin-related CAMs have structures resembling immunoglobulins, but do not represent a 'close' family)'. The structure of these CAMs resembles that of immunoglobulin molecule (Fig.) and it is considered likely that these CAMs later evolved into immunoglobulins during evolution. It is for this reason, that these glycoproteins are called 'immunoglobulin superfamily CAMs'.

Immunoglobulin-related: CAMs were first discovered in *Dictyostelium* (also called a slime mold) which is a unicellular organism (called myxamoeba to distinguish it from true amoeba), that aggregates into multicellular organisation, when starved. This multicellular organisation is facilitated by CAMs. Using antibodies specific to a particular class of CAMs, the presence of these CAMs (a 24-kD glycoprotein) was shown, not in vegetatively dividing cells, but in cells preparing to aggregate.

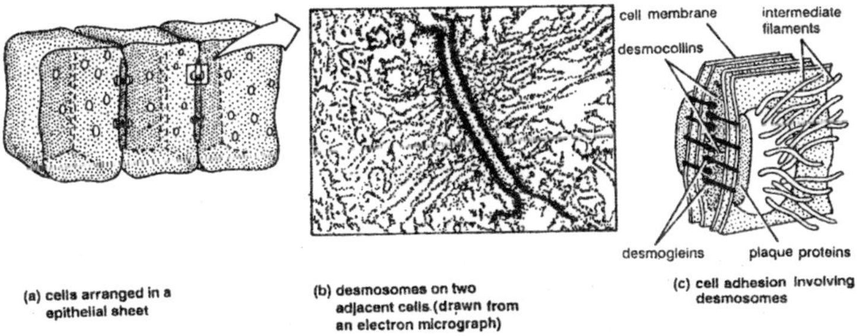

Desmosomes and their involvement in cell adhesion in epidermis (redrawn from Gilbert, 1994).

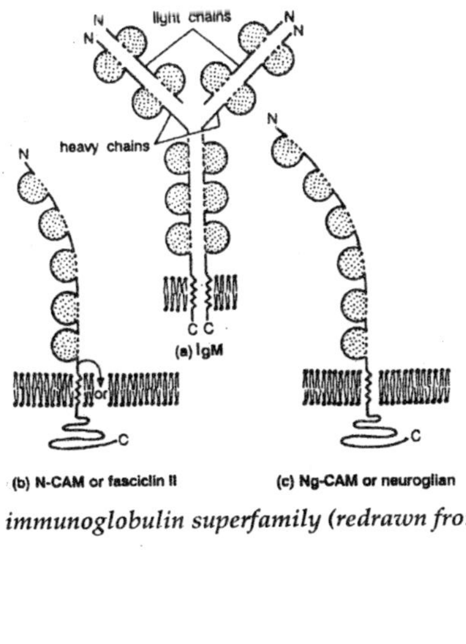

Three members of the immunoglobulin superfamily (redrawn from Gilbert, 1994).

It was also noticed that when antigen binding sites (Fab's) were isolated from antibodies and used with aggregation-competent cells, these cells could not aggregate, due to blocking action of isolated Fab's. (The use of isolated Fab's was necessary, because the whole antibody molecule has two antigen binding sites permitting cross-linking leading to aggregation, even when CAMs react with antibody). Further, when a 80-kD glycoprotein (another CAM) gene was made to express in vegetatively dividing cells, these cells adhered to one another even in vegetative phase (although in vegetative phase they should not adhere). This led to the discovery of a 80-kD glycoprotein that mediates cell-cell adhesion during a slime mold aggregation. The same approach was used in chick embryos to isolate a 140-kD neural cell adhesion molecule or N-CAM, which was shown to play an important role in neuronal aggregation.

Neural cell adhesion molecules (N-CAM) are the most abundant and the best studied example of 'immunoglobulin superfamily CAMs'. They are found in a variety of cell types including nerve cells and bind adjoining cells together by homophilic binding (like cadherins), although there are other Ig-like CAMs, which use heterophilic binding (Fig.). These other Ig like CAMs (involving heterophilic binding) include intercellular adhesion molecules (ICAMs), which are found on activated endothelial cells and bind to integrins (occurring on the surface of white blood cells) to help trapping of white blood cells at the sites of inflammation.

There are atleast 20 forms of N-CAMs, generated by alternative splicing of an RNA transcript produced from a single gene (different cadherins, however, are each encoded by a separate gene). Each N-CAM may consist of (i) extracellular domain folded into five Ig-like domains, (ii) a transmembrane domain spanning the membrane, and (iii) intracellular or cytoplasmic domain, which varies in size and is involved in cell signaling or binding to the cytoskeleton. Some variants of

N-CAMs are shown in Figure and it is obvious that some N-CAMs have extracellular domain only (as a part of ECM), while others are attached to plasma membrane by a glycosylphosphatidyl- inositol (GPI) molecule and still others, having all the three domains, differ in the size of intracellular domain and/or in the degree of glycosylation. N-CAMs also differ in the quantity of associated sialic acid.

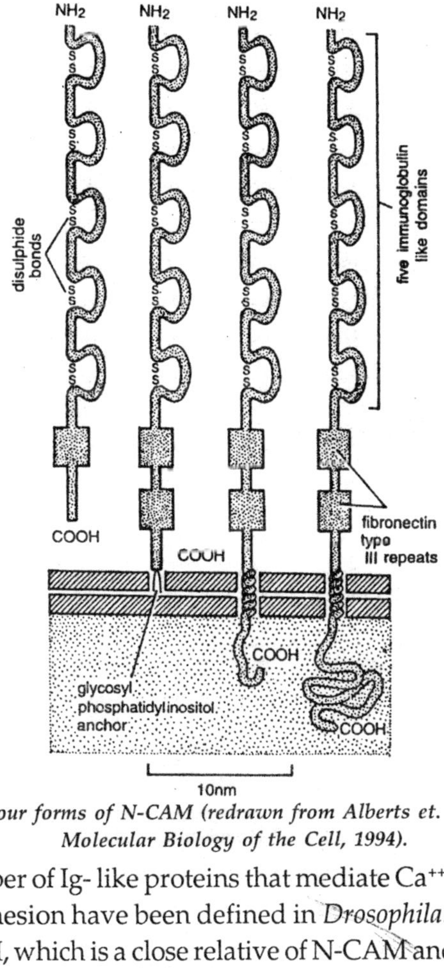

Four forms of N-CAM (redrawn from Alberts et. al., Molecular Biology of the Cell, 1994).

A number of Ig- like proteins that mediate Ca^{++} independent cell-cell adhesion have been defined in *Drosophila*. One of them is fasciclin II, which is a close relative of N-CAM and is expressed on a subset of nerve cell processes and on some of the glial cells. N-CAM and other members of Ig family seem to contribute more to the regulation of cell-cell adhesion interactions during development and regeneration. In contrast to this, cadherins mediate adhesions which are much stronger, playing a major role in binding cells together in tissues and maintaining their integrity.

Role of sialic acid in cell-cell adhesion using N-CAMs. N-CAMs interact homophilically in adjoining cells and make bonds leading to cell-cell adhesion. N-CAMs and N-cadherins are often found on the same cells, but in different regions .

The adhesiveness of the cells with N-CAM molecules can be modified by the amount of sialic acid, so that the cells with low amount of sialic acid on their N-CAMs aggregate four times more readily than those with the high level of sialic acid. As the embryo gets older, most of N-CAM proteins progress from high sialic acid to low sialic acid forms, which may stabilise mature tissues. It has been shown that if two neighbouring cells both express low sialic acid form of N-CAMs, strong cell adhesion is promoted, while in cells containing high sialic acid N-CAMs, cell adhesion is weakened or inhibited (Fig.).

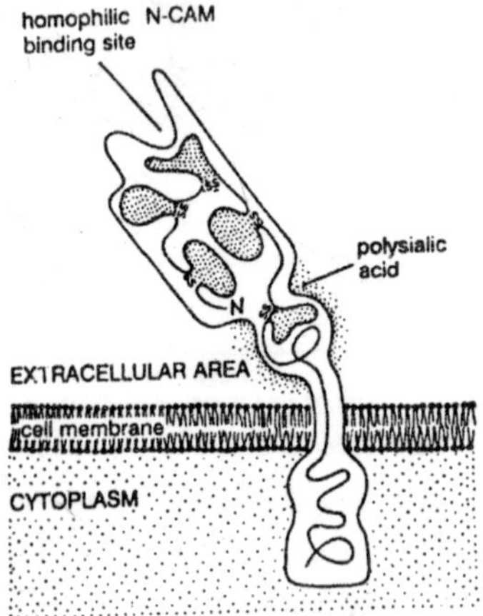

(a) structure of N-CAM molecule

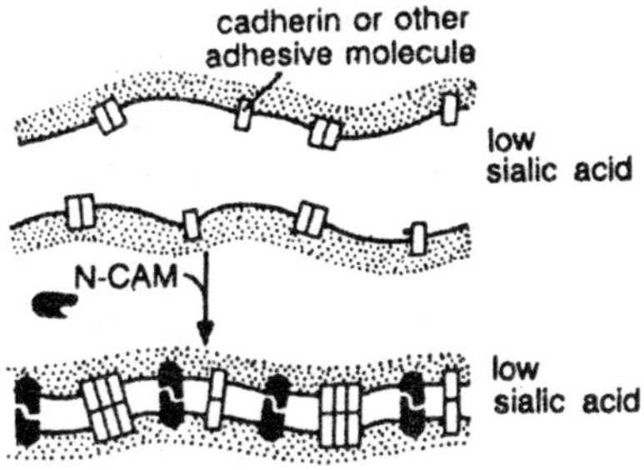

(b) low sialic acid N-CAM molecules and cadherins in cell adhesion

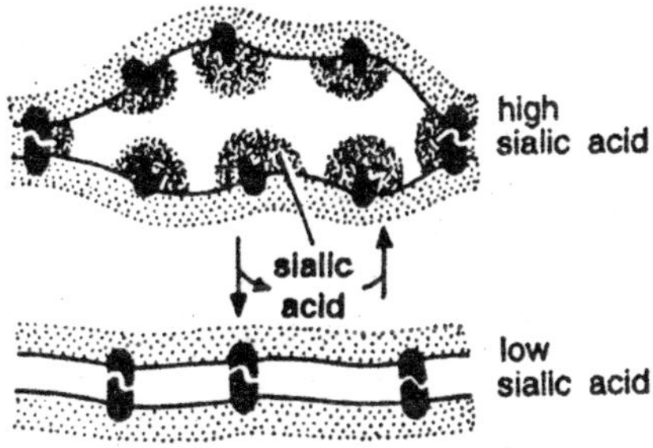

(c) high sialic acid N-CAM molecules in cell adhesion

Mechanism of cell-cell adhesion with the help of N-CAM, involving sialic acid (redrawn from Gilbert, 1994).

Segregation and Binding of Different Cell Types: Segregation of different kinds of cells is also achieved by the presence of different CAMs on these different kinds of cells. For instance, notochord cells do not enter into the neural tube, and dermal cells do not enter epidermis, due to the presence of different CAMs.

Development of feathers in chicken is another example of segregation and adhesion of cells due to CAMs. The ectodermal cells are linked together by E-cadherin, and mesenchymatous cells with N-CAMs form a feather.

CAMs also play a role in binding one cell type to another. For instance, connections between an axon (axons are extensions of nerve cell body and transmit impulses to the target tissues) and its specific target organ is facilitated by N-CAMs.

Furthermore, axons travelling in the same direction bind together due to the presence of same type of CAMs, and form a nerve, a phenomenon called fasciculation. These CAMs may differ at different sites along the length of axons and have been called 'fasciculins', some of which belong to immunoglobulin superfamily.

Selectins: 'Selectins' (name used for the first time by Bevilacqua *et. al.*, 1991) represent a family of three cell surface glycoproteins, that contain lectin domains for recognising cell-specific glycoproteins (found on the surface of some cells) during regional inflammation.

Therefore, the discovery of these selectins has given a meaning to the presence of cell-specific carbohydrates, which are utilised by leukocytes for cell- cell adhesion.

The selectins actually provide for a mechanism of cell-cell (leukocycte-endothelial cell) adhesion, where lectin or carbohydrate recognition domain (CRD) in a selectin of one cell recognises a cell surface carbohydrate of another cell. (This is unlike CAMs, because although like CAMs, they facilitate adhesion, but unlike CAMs, they encourage segregation of cell types).

Following are the three known selectins (Fig.):

(i) L-selectin or leucocyte-selectin (earlier also named as homing receptor, because it is involved in homing of lymphocytes back to the sites from which they were derived) is a 90 to l00kD antigen, confined to leukocyte cell surfaces, and synthesized constitutively.

(ii) E-selectin or endothelial-selectin (earlier also called ELAM-1 or endothelial leukocyte adhesion molecule), located on endothelium, has a molecular mass of 95-115kD and is synthesized within hours on induction of endothelial cells by inflammatory stimuli like interleukin-1 or tumour necrosis factor; this selectin functions as an adhesion molecule and binds neutrophils and monocytes to endothelial cell surface.

(iii) P-selectin or platelet-selectin (earlier also called GMP140 or granule membrane protein of molecular mass 140kD) is also called PADGEM protein (platelet activation-dependent granule external membrane protein).

It is also involved in binding of neutrophils or monocytes to endothelial cell surface, but is stored in platelet alpha granules or endothelial cell Weibel-Palade Bodies. It is induced within minutes (does not take hours as in case of E-selectin) by activation of cells with thrombotic stimuli.

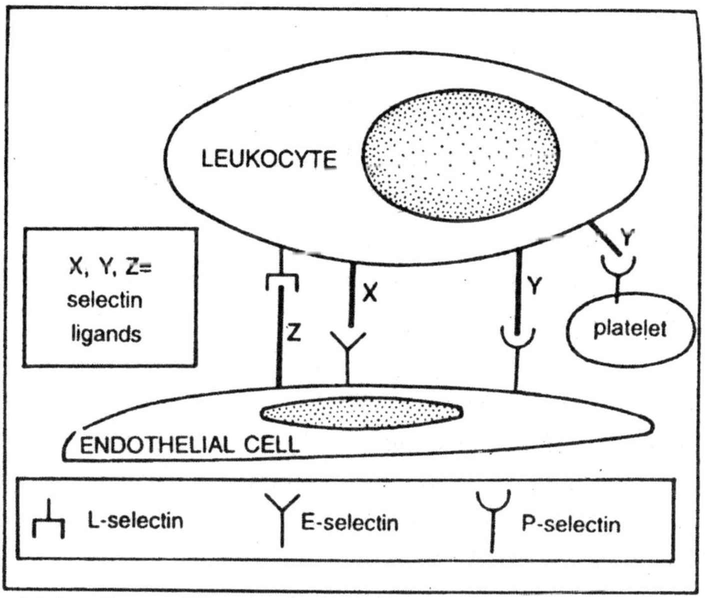

(a) location and topology of the three types of selectins

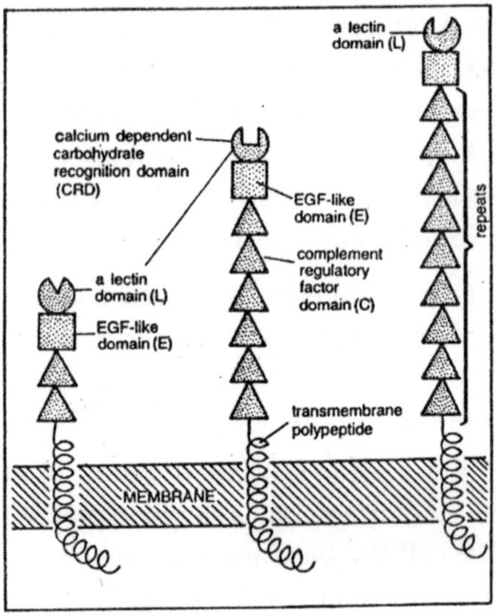

(b) molecular architecture of the three types of selectins

Three types of selectins.

Detailed studies of the above three selectins suggested excellent correspondence between the domain structure of these glycoproteins and the exon-intron structure of the genes encoding them.

The domains in these selectins included the following:

(i) a lectin domain (L) or carbohydrate recognition domain (CRD) for recognition of cell surface carbohydrate (CSC),

(ii) an epidermal growth factor (EGF)—like motif (E) juxtaposed to lectin, and

(iii) a variable number of repetitive domains of glycoprotein C, specific to a selectin and similar to those in various complement binding proteins.

It was shown that the overall similarity of L and E domains of the three selectins was high (65%), while the repetitive C domains were less conserved. The details of the three selectins are summarised in Table.

Some Characteristic Features of Selectins.

Type	*Location*	*Expression*	*Adherent cell types*	*Proposed function*
1. L-selectin (homing receptor)	Leucocytes (constitutive)	Decreases on cell activation	PLN endothelium; endothelium near inflammatory sites	Lymphocyte recirculation through PLN; neutrophil (+ other leucocytes) inflammation
2. E-selectin (ELAM)	Endothelium (transcriptionally activated)	Increases on inflammation (within hours)	Monocytes, neutrophils, T-cell subsets (Th1, Th2)	Leukocyte inflammation
3. P-selectin (GMP 140)	Platelets (α -granules); endothelium (Weibel-Palade Bodies)	Increases upon thrombin activation, histamine, etc. (within minutes)	Monocytes, neutrophils, T cell subsets (Th1, Th2)	Leukocyte inflammation

PLN = peripheral lymph node

Integrins (Cell Receptors for ECM Molecules), Focal Adhesions and Hemidesmosomes: Integrins (so named by Horwitz *et. al.*, 1986 and Tamkun *et. al.*, 1986) are a class of transmembrane adhesion-receptor proteins, so called because they integrate the extracellular and intracellular scaffolds. They are the best characterised extracellular matrix (ECM) receptors.

The ECM proteins on the substratum taking part in adhesion are substrate adhesion molecules and are represented by proteins like fibronectin and vitronectin, while the intracellular scaffold is represented by actin filament bundles (stress bundles). These integrins are present in plasma membrane regions called focal adhesions, which are closely adherent to the substratum (separated by only 10nm-15nm).

The number of focal adhesions is inversely proportional to the rate of movement of the cell on the substratum (ECM). Each integrin has two non-covalently linked α and β subunits, and thus represents a family of transmembrane α β heterodimers.

There are atleast 14 different a subunits (120-180kD), atleast eight different β subunits (90-1 l0kD) and atleast 20 different α β heterodimers. Many of the possible 112 (14 X 8) α β heterodimers are not known *in vivo.* Different heterodimers enable the cells to bind specific extracellular molecules to allow cell-cell and cell-ECM interactions. The integrins are divided into families based upon the β chain component. The largest integrin subfamily is the β_1 or VLA (very late activation antigen) integrins.

There are seven different a subunits (α_1, to α_6, α_v), that share a common β chain. Four of the β_1 integrins bind to laminin. Of these β_1 integrins, α_2 β_1 binds to collagen and laminin, while α_5 β_1 binds solely to flbronectin (collagen, laminin and fibronectin are components of ECM). The β_2 subfamily consists of the leukocyte receptors LFA-1 (α_1 β_2),

MAC-1 ($\alpha_M \beta_2$, CD11b/CD18, Mo-1, CR3) and gpl50,95 ($\alpha_x \beta_2$). LFA-1, is involved in leukocyte/leukocyte or leuckocyte/ endothelial cell or monocyte/endothelial cell interactions. MAC-1 is found on monocytes, neutroblasts and some lymphocytes. Little is known about gp150,95. The β_3 integrin subfamily consists of the platelet glycoprotein IIb/IIIa ($\alpha_{IIb} \beta_3$), fibrinogen receptor and the vitronectin receptor $\alpha_v \beta_3$ (vitronectin is a multifunctional glycoprotein found in circulation tissue, amniotic fluid and urine; it helps to link cell adhesion, defence and cell invasion).

Although both α and β subunits of integrins are needed for binding to fibronectin or laminin, and the focal adhesion structure is controlled from both sides of the membrane, only the β subunit connects with internal cytoskeleton. The interactions among different proteins at focal adhesion appear to be complex as illustrated in Figure. Cytoplasmic domain of β_1 subunit binds α'talin' (215-235kD) and 'α-actinin' (90-100kD). Talin also binds to 'vinculin', which in its turn binds to 'paxillin' and to the COOH-end of 'α-actinin'. The NH_2-end of actinin is bound to 'zyxin' (82kD), and 'actin'. The protein 'tensin' (150-200kD) also binds vinculin and the actin filament. Another family of proteins associated with actin filament includes radixin, ezrin and moesin (REM). Other associated proteins are tenuin and VASP (vasodilator—stimulated phosphoprotein).

It has been shown through the use of antibodies (antibodies would conjugate with specific proteins and will thus control their activity), that most of the above cytoskeleton proteins (present at focal adhesions) are important for adhesions to the substratum or for movements of fibroblasts, etc. These proteins include α-actinin, talin, vinculin, etc. Several protein kinases including $ppl25^{FAK}$ (125 kD focal adhesion kinase) and $pp60^{src}$ are also involved in integrin mediated tyrosine phosphorylation, which seems to be necessary for establishment of focal adhesions or cell-substratum adhesions.

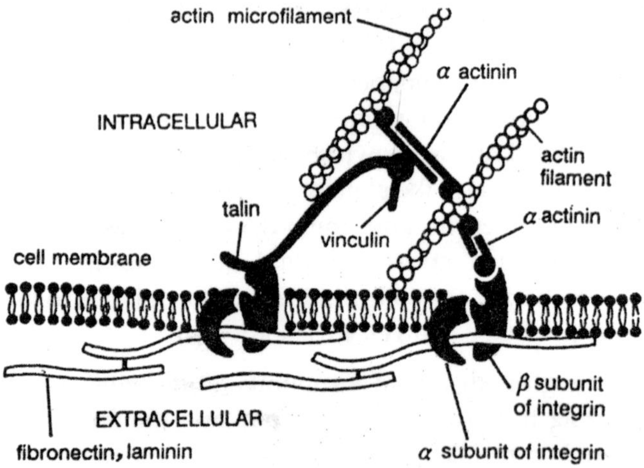

Function of integrins in binding to extracellular matrix (ECM) and the internal cytoskeleton (redrawn from Gilbert, 1994).

Integrins also play an important role during development through tissue and cell adhesion, where one tissue may be used as a substratum for another tissue/cells. Two integrins PS1 and PS2 help in the development of *Drosophila* wing having two epithelial sheets, which are brought together by these integrins.

Integrins, anchorage dependence and anoikis. Most cells in tissues are attached to one another and to the ECM. Only the cells circulating in the blood are designed to survive without attachment and spreading.

The above attachment of cells with other cells and to the ECM and their subsequent spreading on the ECM substrate is essential for proper growth, function and even survival of these cells. Without this attachment and spreading, cells often die and undergo programmed cell death (PCD) or apoptosis. This dependence of cell growth and survival on substrate attachment is known as anchorage dependence and the apoptosis resulting from lack of anchorage is described as anoikis.

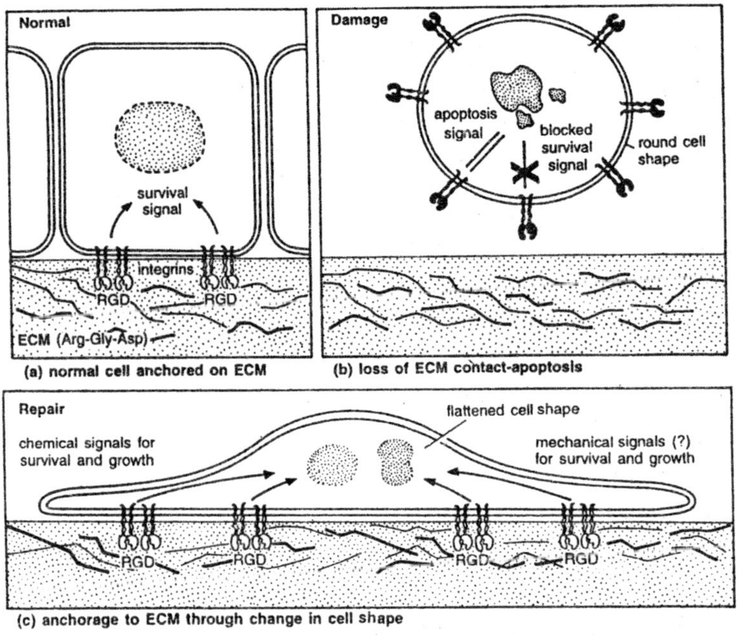

Role of integrins in anchorage dependence and its relationship with cell shape and cell survival.

Integrins play an important role in anchorage dependence and anoikis. Besides linking structural elements, these integrins also trigger a number of signaling pathways. For instance integrins activate many signaling molecules including Ras-Faf-mitogen activated kinase, protein kinase C and phosphatidylinositol 3' kinase. Several integrins utilise focal adhesion kinase (FAK) enzyme for control of anchorage dependence, so that a mutant form of this enzyme, which does not require integrins and cell attachment for its activity, can render cells independent of anchorage. It has also been shown that the biochemical signals originating from ECM-bound integrins are responsible for anchorage-dependent survival and growth of cells.

Another feature that regulates anchorage dependence is cell shape. It is known that flattened cells thrive better than rounded cells. More recently (in 1997), it was shown in a study that the cells forced to extend themselves over a larger surface area survive better and proliferate faster than the cells with a rounded shape. It was also shown that while ECM controls cell shape, cell shape in turn controls survival and growth. This involves activation of certain pathways and inactivation of some other pathways.

For instance in flattened and well spread cells, integrins mediate signals for survival, while in the rounded cells, these survival signals are blocked and apoptosis signals are activated. Similarly in the damaged tissue, fewer cells that will cover the damaged area, will be able to spread to larger surface area, thus stimulating proliferation until the tissue gap is filled (Fig.).

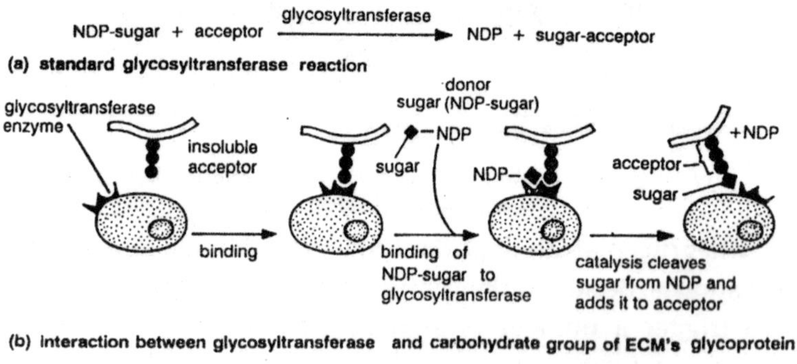

Interaction between glycosyltransferase, carbohydrate and peptides in the extracellular matrix (ECM) to form glycoprotein of ECM. (redrawn from Gilbert, 1994).

Glycosyltransferases (Cell Receptors for ECM Molecules): Glycosyltransferases is another class of cell membrane proteins that help in adhesion of cells to ECM (like integrins). These enzymes are routinely found in the endoplasmic reticulum and Golgi vesicles, where they add sugar residues to peptides forming glycoproteins (Fig.). Different glycosyltransferases are meant for adding different sugars. For instance, galactosyltransferases are meant for transfer of galactose from UDP-galactose to an acceptor.

The glycosyltransferases of plasma membrane recognise the carbohydrate acceptors on the ECM proteins such as laminin leading to adhesion. When the second substrate (*e.g.*, UDP-galactose or NDP-sugar) appears, the adhesions can be broken by the catalysis.

Glycosyltransferases also help in fertilization, where galactosyltransferase on the sperm cell membrane interacts with the carbohydrate components of ECM secreted by the egg, but no catalysis occurs. Glycosyltransferases are also involved in migration of cells, where sugar is transferred to the substrate on which cells migrate.

Union of Cell

Specialised junctions are found in all animal tissues among cells of a tissue and between cells and ECM to allow for cell-cell and cell-matrix contacts. They are particularly abundant and important in epithelia.

Cell junctions are also found in plants and are described there as plasmodesmata. These cell cell junctions and cell-matrix junctions are collectively called cell junctions and can be of the following three functional types:

(i) occluding junctions, which seal cells together in an epithelial sheet preventing the passage of even small molecules from one side of the sheet to the other;

(ii) anchoring junctions, which allow attachment of cells to their neighbouring cells or to ECM and

(iii) communicating junctions, which allow the chemical or electrical signals to pass from one cell to another. These three types of junctions, and particularly the anchoring and communicating junctions are further classified into subclasses, depending upon the location and function of these cell junctions.

Different Types of Cell Junctions.

(1) Occluding junctions (tight junctions)

(2) Anchoring junctions

  (a) Actin filament attachment sites

    (i) cell-cell adherens junctions (*e.g.*, adhesion belts)

    (ii) cell matrix adherens junctions (*e.g.*, focal contacts)

    (iii) septate junctions (invertebrates only)

  (b) Intermediate filament attachment sites

    (i) cell-cell adhesion (desmosomes)

    (ii) cell-matrix adhesion (hemi-desmosomes)

(3) Communicating junctions

  (a) gap junctions

  (b) chemical synapses

  (c) plasmodesmata (plants only)

Cell Junctions in Animals: Occluding junctions (tight junctions). Occluding junctions or tight junctions between epithelial cells help formation of a sheet like structure, which functions as a selective barrier between fluids on either side of this sheet.

For instance, the epithelial cells lining the mammalian small intestine or gut do not allow most of the contents in the cavity (lumen) to pass on to the other side of the epithelium, but do allow the transport of selected nutrients from the lumen across the epithelium sheet.

After permeating through the connective tissue, these selected nutrients diffuse into blood vessels. This transcellular transport depends on two sets of membrane bound carrier proteins:

(i) carrier proteins confined to apical surface (surface facing the lumen) actively transport (Na^+- driven glucose symport) selected molecules from lumen into the cells and

(ii) carrier proteins confined to basolateral surface allow passage of molecules from the cell to extracellular fluid by facilitated diffusion (by glucose carriers). In view of the different mechanisms involved in transport from apical surface and basolaferal surface, the carrier proteins should not be allowed to migrate from one area to another, and the spaces between epithelial cells are sealed, so that the transported molecules do not diffuse back from intercellular spaces (Fig.). Permeability of different epithelia to small molecules differs, so that the epithelium lining the small intestine is 10,000 times more permeable to inorganic ions (*e.g.*, Na^+) than the epithelium lining the urinary bladder.

The tight junctions have been shown to consist of an anastomosing network of strands, each composed of long rows of specific transmembrane proteins in each of the two interacting plasma membranes, which join to occlude the intercellular space.

Anchoring Junctions: Anchoring junctions are widely distributed in animal cells, their function being performed by plasmodesmata in plant cells. They help in connecting cytoskeletal elements of one cell either to the cytoskeletal elements of another cell (cell-cell adherens junctions) or to ECM (cell-matrix adherens junctions). They are most common in tissues like heart muscle or skin epithelium, which are subjected to mechanical stress. These anchoring junctions include:

(i) adherens junctions (connection sites for actin filaments), and

(ii) desmosomes and hemidesmosomes (connection sites for intermediate filaments). They are composed of two

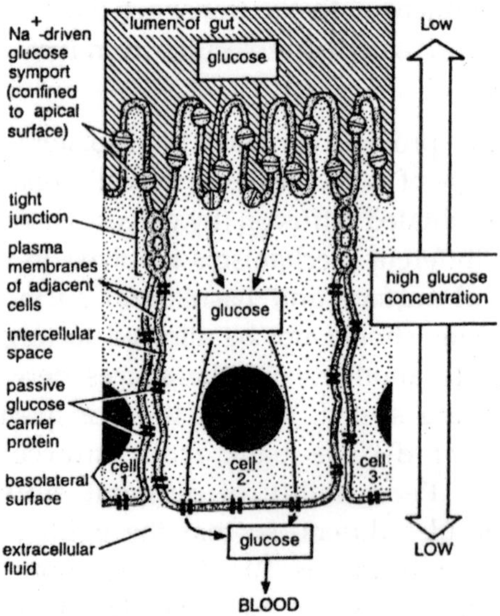

The role of tight junctions in transcellular transport (redrawn from Alberts et. al., Molecular Biology of the Cell, 1994).

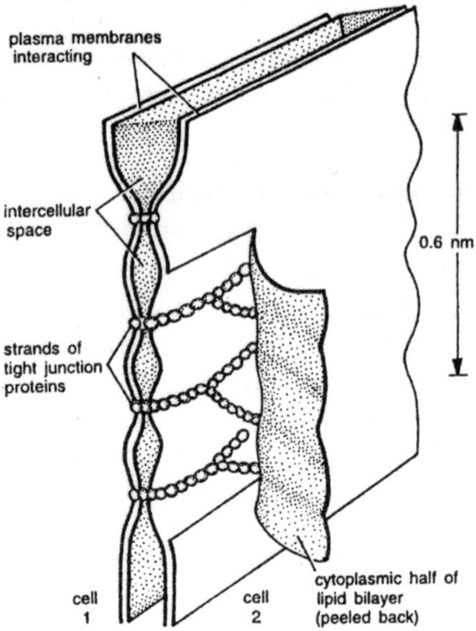

A model of a tight junction (redrawn from Alberts et. al., Molecular Biology of the Cell, 1994).

types of proteins, namely intracellular attachment proteins and transmembrane linker proteins like cadherins and integrins (Table). The cytoplasmic domain of a transmembrane linker protein binds to one or more intracellular attachment proteins, while its extracellular domain interacts either with the extracellular matrix or with the extracellular domain of the transmembrane linker protein of an adjoining cell (Fig.). Septate junctions are also anchoring junctions but they are unique to invertebrates and function as connecting sites for actin filaments, although rarely they can also function as permeability barriers. Much less is known about these septate junctions. The details of the different proteins and cytoskeletal elements involved in anchoring junctions are listed in Table.

Transmembrance and Intracellular Proteins along with Cytoskeletal Elements Involved in Different Anchoring Proteins (Modified from Alberts et. al., 1994).

Anchoring junction	*Transmembrane linker protein*	*Extracellular ligand attachment*	*Intracellular cytoskeletal proteins*	*Intracellular attachment*
1. Adherens (cell-cell)	Cadherin (E-cadherin)	Cadherin in neighbouring cell	Actin filaments	Catenins, vinculin, α-actinin, plakoglobin
2. Desmosomes	Cadherin (desmogleins & desmocollins)	Cadherin in neighbouring cell	Intermediate filaments	Desmoplakins, plakoglobin
3. Adherens (cell-matrix)	Integrin	ECM proteins	Actin filaments	Talin, vinculin, α-actinin
4. Hemi-desmosomes	Integrin ($\alpha_6\beta_4$)	ECM proteins (basal lamina)	Intermediate filaments	Desmoplakin like protein

Communicating Junctions: As shown in Table, communicating junctions meant for passage of chemical or electrical substances (*e.g.* ions) include gap junctions, chemical synapses and plasmodesmata. Gap junctions and chemical synapses are common in animals, while plasmodesmata are the only intercellular junctions in plants.

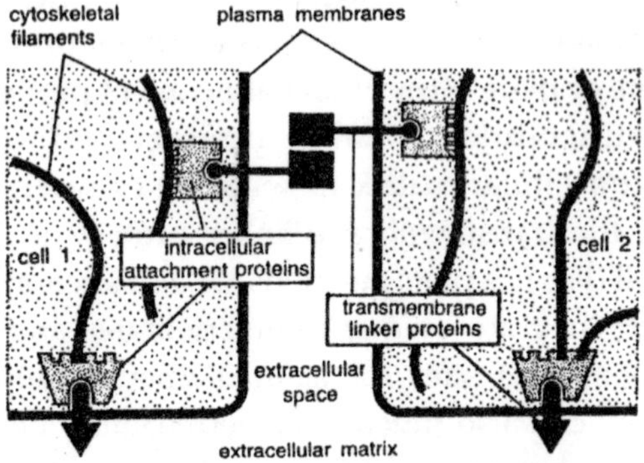

Construction of an anchoring junction with the help of two classes of proteins-intercellular attachment proteins and transmembrane linker proteins (redrawn from Alberts et. al., Molecular Biology of the Cell, 1994).

Gap Junctions in Animals: Cell-cell attachments and communications are also facilitated by certain proteins, forming 'gap junctions' between cells which maintain a gap, 2nm to 4nm wide. In tight junctions, on the other hand, plasma membranes of two cells appear to be in direct contact without any gap. These gap junctions are the most widespread of all cell junctions and are found in all tissues in all animal species.

Under electron microscope, they appear as patches between cells separated by a gap. The ability of cells to form gap junctions with some specific cells and not with others enable the formation of physiological compartments (each compartment with a multitude of cells) within a developing embryo. Antibodies to gap junction proteins, when injected into young embryos have been found to interfere with flow of ions leading to abnormal development.

The gap junction channels are made up of structures called 'connexons', which in their turn, are made up of transmembrane proteins called 'connexins' each, with four membrane spanning α -helices. Six identical connexins group together to form a transmembrane channel (connexon) containing a central pore (lined by one transmembrane helix from each connexin).

When a connexon comes in contact with a similar channel from an adjoining cell, it forms a gap junction providing communication between cytoplasms of the two cells (Fig.). This channel is larger and more permeable than either the neurotransmitter gated channel (with five subunits) or the voltage gated cation channels (with four subunits). Different types of connexins may be regulated by cadherins, so that cadherins not only help in cell adhesion, but also work for modifying the connexin proteins.

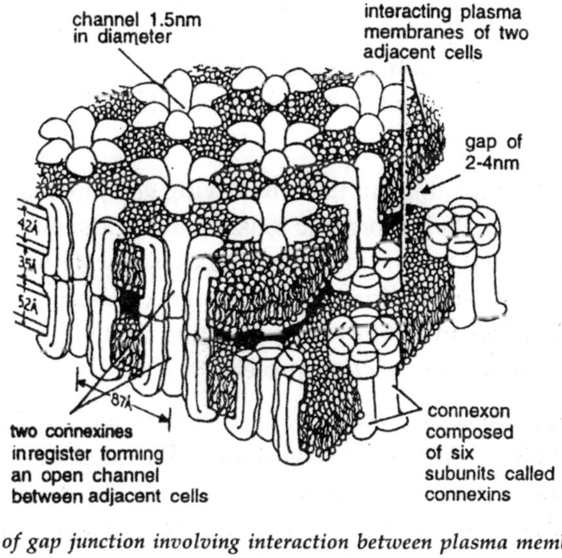

A model of gap junction involving interaction between plasma membranes of two adjacent cells.

In December 1996, at the Sixth International Congress of Cell Biology held at San Francisco, atleast three connexins were shown to be associated with three diseases (in mice and humans). An abnormality in connexin 43 was shown to be associated with defect in the heart of a child; a defect in connexin

37 (which forms junctions between oocytes and the surrounding tissue) led to female infertility in mice and may be associated with premature menopause in human females; and the absence of connexin 46 was shown to be responsible for cataracts in mice.

It was therefore concluded that connexin 43 might play a role in heart development, connexin 37 might allow the right signals to reach the eggs to mature and connexin 46 may be important for maintaining lens transparency in eye. It is speculated that association of many more connexins with more diseases will be discovered in future.

The gap junctions have each a pore (~1.5nm in diameter) and, through this pore, small water soluble molecules (not bigger than 1000 daltons) pass from cytoplasm of one cell to that of another. These cells connected by gap junctions are described as electrically coupled, when ions pass through gap junctions or metabolically coupled, when other micromolecules are involved.

Thus the adjoining animal cells having gap junctions share with each other their inorganic ions, amino acids, nucleotides and vitamins, but not the macromolecules like proteins, nucleic acids and polysaccharides. The passage of these ions and micromolecules can be blocked by injecting antibodies directed against a major gap junction protein.

Gap junctions are found, both in tissues with electrically excitable cells and in those having no such excitable cells. In nerve cells (a class of electrically excitable cells), electrical coupling due to transport of ions through gap junctions, allows action potential to spread rapidly from cell to cell without any delay that occurs at cell synapses. This is useful, where a quick response is needed (*e.g.* escape responses in fish and insects). In tissues with no electrically excitable cells, sharing of metabolites allow *firstly,* the coordination of the activities of cells (*e.g.* beating of cilia) and *secondly,* it eliminates random fluctuations from cell to cell. AMP and Ca^{++} ions can also pass through gap junctions, to allow propagation of responses to extracellular signals.

During embryogenesis (in vertebrates also), cells are electrically coupled due to passage of ions through gap junctions. When cells in embryos start differentiating, they uncouple from surrounding tissues through regulation of passage via gap junctions. For instance, during formation of neural tube from neural plate, its cells uncouple from surrounding tissue.

It is thus obvious that channels formed by gap junction do not always remain open and that the opening of the pore is regulated by changes in pH and Ca^{++} ion concentration. Gap junctions thus are dynamic structures like ion channels and conformational changes in protein subunits forming gap junctions may be involved in opening and closing of these channels (Fig.).

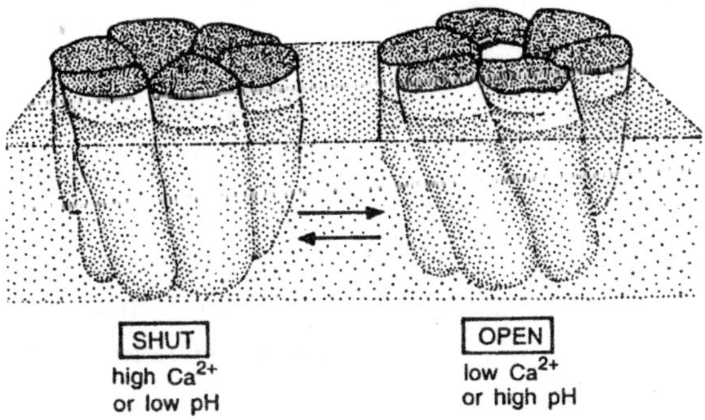

A model showing mechanism for closing of gap junction channel due to rise in Ca^{2+} or fall in pH in the cytosol (redrawn from Alberts et. al., Molecular Biology of the Cell, 1994).

Cell Junctions in Plants

Plasmodesmata: The presence of cell wall in plants though eliminates the need for anchoring junctions to hold the cells in place, but the need for direct cell-cell communication remains.

Only one type of cell junctions are known in plants and these are plasmodesmata (PD), which like gap junctions bring about coupling between cytoplasm of adjoining cells. The plasmodesmata form fine cytoplasmic channels (20-40 nm in diameter) between cells. Running through the centre of this channel is a narrow cylindrical structure called desmotubule, which is continuous with the endoplasmic reticula of adjoining cells. Between the inner wall of plasmodesmata and the desmotubule, is a cytosolic annulus through which molecules can pass (Fig.).

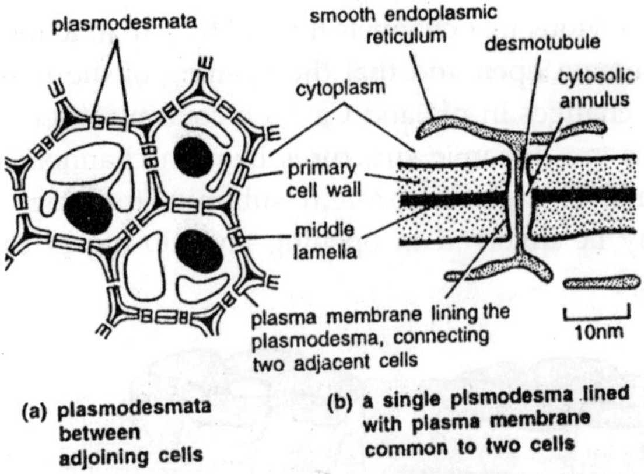

Structure of plasmodesmata (redrawn from Alberts et. al., Molecular Biology of the Cell, 1994).

The plasmodesmata resemble gap junctions in many ways. However in contrast to these gap junctions in animals, plasmodesmata in plants are elongated structures traversing the thick cell walls. Each PD has:

(i) an outer sheath contiguous with the plasma membrane,

(ii) a central core of endoplasmic reticulum (ER) and

(iii) a collar or neck region.

Plasmodesmata (PD) are known for long and were initially assigned a passive role of permitting free movements of small metabolites and growth hormones (less than 1 kilodalton) between plant cells. Later, when it was found that large genomes of plant viruses could traverse from one cell to another, it was suggested that viruses alter the PD to allow transport of very large molecules like viral genomes.

More recent work, however, suggests that plasmodesmata are not meant for a mere passive role as above, but are rather dynamic structures, rapidly altering their dimensions to allow transport of bigger molecules, like viral genomes and endogenous plant proteins. It has also been shown recently that the macromolecules track through the plant cytoplasm with the help of cytoskeleton, which functions as a major tracking system to the site of PD.

Movement proteins (MP) of plant viruses have been discovered, which operate an endogenous PD transport system. If MP is injected into single cells, the permeability of PD is increased within minutes of microinjection, confirming this role of MP. It has also been shown that PDs in different cell types in plants are diverse and therefore, respond differently to MP in different cell types.

For instance, in tobacco leaves, in the absence of MP the plasmodesmata in trichome hair cell allow transport of molecules less than 7 kD and those in the mesophyll cells allow transport of molecules less than 1 kD.

However, MP induced gating permits movement of dextrans (more than 20 kD) in mesophyll cells, but not in trichome cells, although MP itself (30 kD) moves in both cell types. It has also been shown that a 30 kD MP mediates movement of a 68 kD reporter protein, when present in cis-orientation with MP, but not when present in trans-orientation (*i.e.* not transported unless attached with MP).

This suggests that MP has a transport signal which dictates transport irrespective of the size of the molecule to be transported. The four criteria for a molecule to be transported include size, shape, signal sequence and gating junction. The structure and behaviour of PD itself depends on cell/tissue type and the developmental stage.

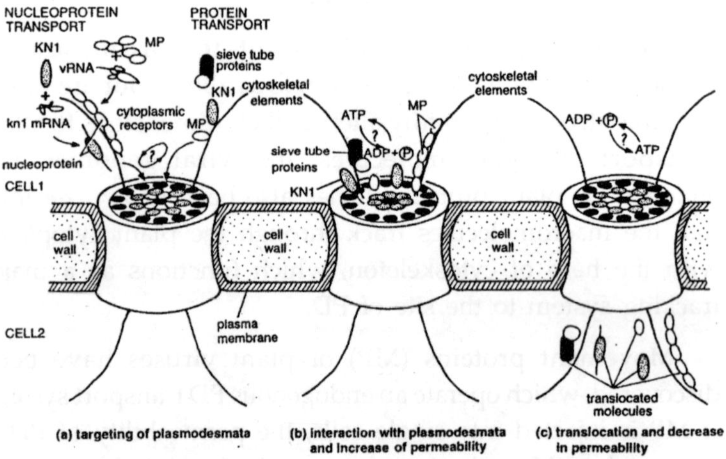

Translocation of various nucleoproteins and proteins through plasmodesmata.

Intercellular transport of RNA and protein molecules through PD in maize has been inferred by locating the presence of RNA and protein molecules encoded by specific genes. For instance, during development, RNA transcribed by *knl* gene is not found in outermost L1 layer of meristem, but the *knl* gene encoded KN1 (KNOTTED 1) protein (a transcription factor) is found in this layer suggesting that this must have been transported through PD from other cells, where RNA is present and gets translated into protein.

KN1 protein not only moves between mesophyll cells but also facilitates movement of dextrans and proteins larger than 20 kD. KN1 protein also selectively transports *knl* sense RNA but not antisense RNA between cells.

Such regulation of the movement of molecules by regulation of the distribution and permeability of PD may actually regulate development and differentiation. Plasmodesmata are also implicated in the movement of numerous proteins (upto as large as 70 kD) from companion cells to the enucleate sieve elements of the phloem.

Another aspect relevant to the function of PD is the mechanism of movement of molecules within the cytoplasm to reach PD. In this connection, co-localisation of MP with microtubules and actin filaments and its involvement in transport through PD (as shown above) suggest that the cytoskeleton is used for tracking of macromolecules to PD.

The cytoskeleton may also be involved in gating of PD. Actin filaments also traverse PD channels and actin may act as sphincter at the neck region of PD. Additional cellular factors may interact with actin to generate an open/closed PD conformation thus regulating transport.

8

Demise of Cell

Development and homeostasis in most multicellular organisms are dependent on cell division, differentiation and cell death. During development, the interaction between the processes of cell division and cell death leads to the generation of proper numbers and types of cells. In a mature animal also, a balance (homeostasis) is maintained between different types of cells due to a critical balance between cell division and cell death. Almost 50 years ago (around the year 1950), it was established that cells die as a normal part of development and homeostasis. This deliberate elimination of unwanted cells in a morphologically distinct manner (cells shrink and get phagocytosed) is described as programmed cell death (PCD) or apoptosis, as against the pathological cell death caused due to cell injury (cells swell and burst to release toxins).

Naturally-occurring programmed cell death is found in all animals, although its detailed analysis has been conducted only in some animal systems (in the nematode, *Coenorhabditis elegans* cell death has been most extensively studied). In vertebrates, cell death has been observed in all developing tissues and has been most extensively studied in the developing nervous system and immune system. Like nematodes, in invertebrates also, cell death occurs in many tissues during development, including neurons, muscle cells, epithelial cells, intestinal cells and gonadal cells.

Cell death or apoptosis has also been observed in microbial systems/cell cultures and therefore is ubiquitous. Alterations in the programmed cell death leading to survival of those cells which were targeted to undergo cell death has also been found to cause a number of human diseases.

For instance, if the cells destined for cell death survive in mutants, it may lead to cancer or autoimmune diseases, while excessive cell death may cause neurodegenerative disease and immunodeficiency (autoimmune disease means immunity against one's own cells or its constituents). In view of this, cell death or apoptosis has been an area of intensive research in recent years.

The execution of programmed cell death (PCD) or apoptosis is often associated with characteristic morphological and biochemical changes. During this process, the nucleus and the cytoplasm condense, and the dying cell is broken into membrane-bound apoptotic pieces, which are rapidly engulfed (or phagocytosed) and digested by macrophages or by neighbouring cells.

Thus the dead cells are removed and any harm due to leakage of their dangerous contents is avoided. On the other hand, in the pathological death due to injury, cells swell and lyse thus releasing cytoplasmic material causing inflammation (Fig.). Apoptosis is also associated with the activation of nucleases and also with the synthesis of RNA and proteins, so that it is a gene directed active process, which is regulated in a precise manner. The following aspects of apoptosis, utilising suitable examples, will be discussed in this chapter: (i) the role which this process of apoptosis plays in differentiation and

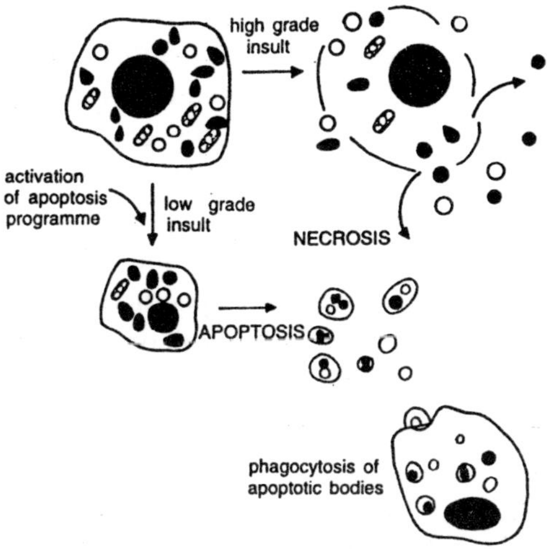

A comparison between programmed cell death (PCD) or apoptosis and pathological death (necrosis, due to high grade insult) (redrawn from Cotter and Al-Rubeai, TIBTECH, April 1995).

development, (ii) the specific genes which are involved in this process, (iii) the mechanism of its occurrence and the manner in which this process is regulated.

Apoptosis in Coenorhabditis Elegans: The phenomenon of cell death or apoptosis has been most extensively studied in the nematode, C. *elegans*, which has become the most suitable organism for the developmental studies due to the following two reasons. *Firstly*, being transparent, cell divisions or cell deaths can be observed easily in this organism, and *secondly*, the availability of the detailed data on genetic and molecular analysis makes the dissection of the various aspects of cell death easily approachable.

The adult nematode is a male or a hermaphrodite, which has 1090 somatic cells, which are formed during development; 131 of these 1090 cells undergo programmed cell death (PCD), which is precisely controlled, so that in every animal, the same cells at the same characteristic time will die. Programmed cell death in *C. elegans* can be divided into the following four distinct stages shown in Figure: (i) decision of whether a cell will die or survive (cell death specificity); (ii) the execution of cell death; (iii) the engulfment of dead cells by phagocytes and (iv) degradation of the engulfed corpses. Mutations affecting each of these four stages have been isolated and genes controlling all these stages identified. In all, there are following 14 genes already known to control these four stages: *ces-1, ces-2* and *egl-1* controlling cell specificity (stage 1); *ced-3, ced-4* and *ced-9* controlling the cell death (stage-2); *ced-1, ced-2, ced-5, ced-6, ced-7, ced-8* and *ced-10* controlling the engulfment (stage-3) and *nuc-1* controlling the degradation (stage-4).

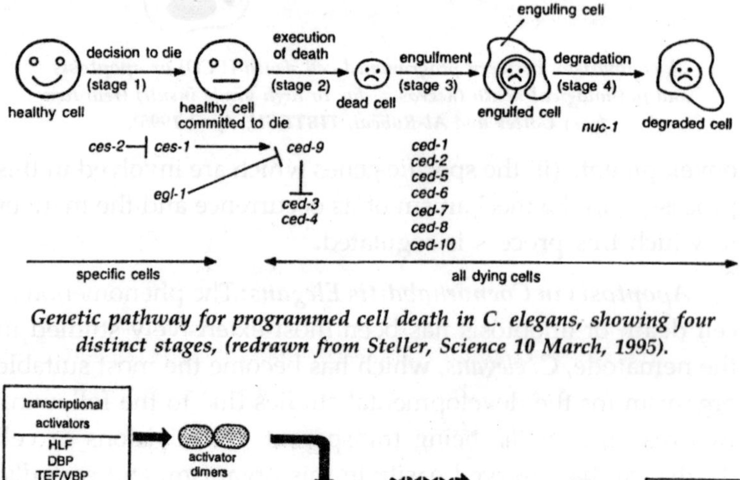

Genetic pathway for programmed cell death in C. elegans, showing four distinct stages, (redrawn from Steller, Science 10 March, 1995).

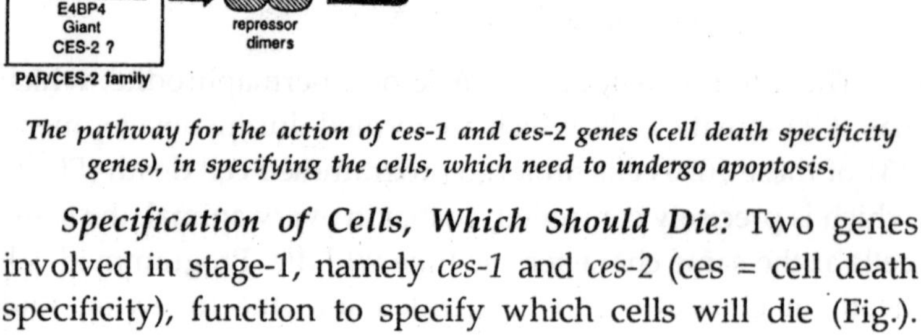

The pathway for the action of ces-1 and ces-2 genes (cell death specificity genes), in specifying the cells, which need to undergo apoptosis.

Specification of Cells, Which Should Die: Two genes involved in stage-1, namely *ces-1* and *ces-2* (ces = cell death specificity), function to specify which cells will die (Fig.).

Dominant mutations in *ces-1* gene prevent death of four neurons in the pharynx and mutation in *ces-2* prevents two of these deaths by negatively regulating *ces-1*. Mutations in the third gene involved in stage-1, *i.e., egl-1* (egl = egg laying) cause the death of two HSN neurons which control egg laying by the hermaphrodite (these two neurons normally die in males, but survive in hermaphrodites).

Actual Death of Specified Cells: Two genes involved in stage-2 of apoptosis, namely *ced-3*, and *ced-4 (ced* = cell death abnormal) have been identified to be responsible for programmed cell death, and mutations in any one of them, leads to survival of almost all cells that would die in the normal individual. In mosaic animals also, cells die in those tissues where active *ced-3* and *ced-4* occur and survive in those which carry a mutation for either of these two genes. Both these genes have been isolated and the DNA sequences for both these genes are now known, suggesting that *ced-4* codes for a protein with Ca^{2+} sites and *ced-3* codes for a protein (a cysteine protease) with phosphorylation sites. The cell death, therefore, may be mediated by Ca^{2+} binding and by protein phosphorylation, although this has not been tested experimentally.

The *ced-3* and *ced-4* appear to be negatively regulated by another gene, *ced-9*, so that dominant *ced-9* mutations may either prevent cell death or may cause lethality to the organism (due to death of cells that would otherwise survive). This gene *(ced-9)* is thus, required to protect cells that should escape undergoing programmed cell death and survive. The gene *ced-9* encodes a protein that is homologous to the Bcl-2 family of cell death regulators encoded by mammalian oncogene *bcl-2* (for Bcl-2, see later).

Engulfment of Cell Corpses: The cells, which die as above are engulfed by neighbouring cells, through what is described as phagocytosis of cell corpses. Seven genes have been identified, such that mutation in any one of them can prevent engulfment of some cell corpses, although most corpses appear to be engulfed normally. In some double mutants, far fewer corpses are engulfed. Mutations in genes *ced-2, ced-5* and *ced-10* cause major defect in engulfment, while mutations in the remaining four genes *(ced-1, ced-6, ced-7* or *ced-8)* cause relatively minor defect.

Degradation of Cell Corpses: The engulfed cell corpses have to undergo degradation under the control of a gene *nuc-1.* Mutation in this gene leads to loss of ability to degrade DNA, so that the pycnotic DNA. persists. The gene *nuc-1* controls an endonuclease enzyme, but unlike mammalian nucleases, this endonuclease does not require Ca^{2+}.

Cell Death in Mammals (Bcl-2 and ICE Proteins or Caspases): In neoplastic (tumorous) tissues, an increase in the number of cells is viewed as a violation of normal homeostasis. This increase in the number of cells is caused either by increased cell division or by decreased cell death. The gene, *bcl-2* is an oncogene on human chromosome 18, and studies of transgenic mice carrying *bcl-2,* showed that *bcl-2* leads to absence of cell death rather than increased cell division. In a common tumour of human B cells (follicular lymphoma), a segment of chromosome 18 carrying the gene *bcl-2* is translocated with a segment of chromosome 14 carrying an immunoglobulin locus.

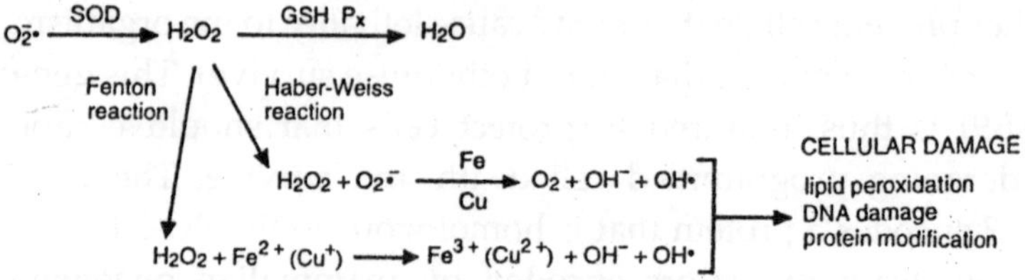

An online showing the manner in which reactive oxygen species (ROS), in the form of hydroxyl radicals (OH*), may be involved in programmed cell death; Bcl-2 blocks this oxidative damage (redrawn from Korsmeyer, TIG, March, 1995).

It has been shown that *bcl-2* expression rescued lymphoid and myeloid cells from an otherwise inevitable death caused by withdrawal of the cytokine interleukin-3. The cells, rescued thus due to *bcl-2* expression, do not proliferate, suggesting that Bcl-2 protein is a true 'survival factor', rather than a mere inhibitor of cell death and differs from mitogens. Later, it was also shown that *bcl-2* expression has a key role to play in the maturation of B-cells in follicle centres, specifying the survival of small minority of cells destined to become memory cells following antigen challenge.

Bcl-2 protein has a carboxy-terminal hydrophobic region localised to mitochondria, endoplasmic reticulum and nuclear membrane, with its amino terminal region facing the cytosol. Lipid membranes are sites where reactive oxygen species (ROS) engage in damage. Bcl-2 blocks such a damage and also blocks gamma-irradiation induced cell death caused due to hydroxyl radicals (OH), which are produced in reactions shown in Figure. It also protects cells from the lethal attacks of H_2O_2, t-butyl hydroperoxide and several other chemicals in a dose dependent manner. At low doses of these chemicals, cell death resembles apoptosis. Two critical amino acids were identified (gly-145 and trp-188), which were essential for Bcl-2's function as a survival factor.

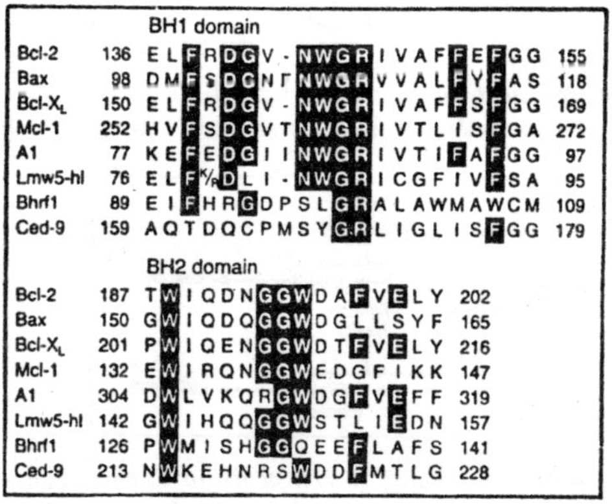

Homologues within the Bcl-2 protein family, highlighting the two homology domains. BH1 and BH2 (amino acids that are identical in members are shown in black boxes (redrawn from Korsmeyer, TIG, March, 1995).

Bcl-2 is a member of multiprotein complex family, which includes (i) a 21kD Bax (Bcl-2 associated X protein), (ii) Bcl-$_{XL}$; (iii) Mcl-1; (iv) Al; (v) Lmw5-hl; (vi) Bhrfl, (vii) Ced-9. They show highest degree of conservation in regions characterised as Bcl-2 homology 1 and 2 (BH1 and BH2) domains (Fig.). Bax remains associated with Bcl-2 and promotes cell death, which is opposed by Bcl-2, so that when Bcl-2 dimers are in excess, cells survive and when Bax dimers are in excess, cells die. Bcl-2 must bind with Bax to exert its effect so that Bcl-2/Bax heterodimers or Bax homodimers regulate cell death. Bcl-2-Bax heterodimers and not the Bcl-2-Bcl-2 homodimers are the active moiety preventing cell death (Fig.). It has also been shown that mutation in either of two essential amino acids mentioned above (gly-145, trp-188) destroy the ability of Bcl-2 to heterodimerise with Bax, to prevent cell death.

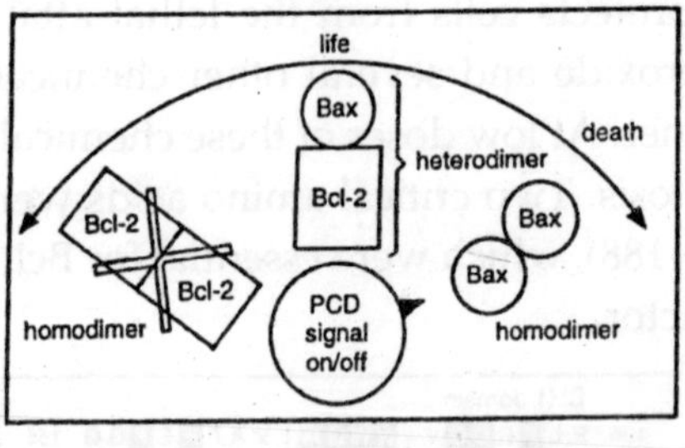

Regulation of cell death in mammals by Bcl-2/Bax heterodimers and Bax-homodimers (redrawn from Korsmeyer, TIG, March, 1995).

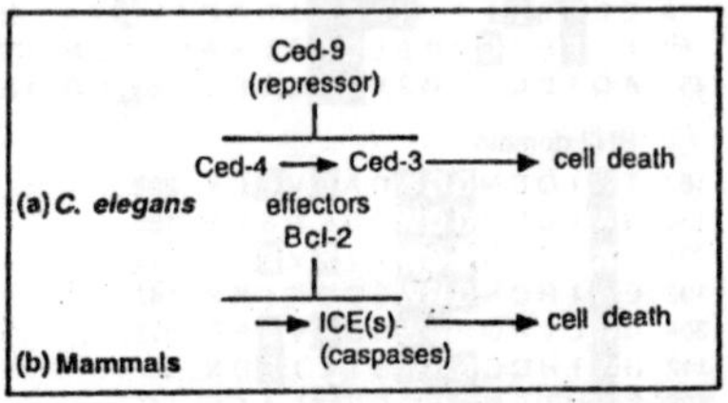

A genetic pathway leading to cell death in C. elegans and in multicellular organisms; ced-3 and ced-4 are effective in cell death, while ced-9 is death repressor in C. elegans; similarly, ICE sequence encoding caspases causes cell death and bcl-2 prevents cell death in multicellular organisms (redrawn from Korsmeyer, TIG, March, 1995).

It has been shown that Ced-9 protein (a repressor) of *C. elegans* is the nematode homologue of Bcl-2 in mammals, having homology in BH1 and BH2 domains. Ced-3 protein of *C. elegans* also has homology to a known mammalian protein, the interleukin-1 β converting enzyme (ICE), which is a cysteine protease with a novel specificity for aspartic acid. More recently, ICEs have been called caspases, whose activation eventually causes cell death. Overexpression of these caspases or Ced-3 causes cell death and overexpression of Bcl-2 or Ced-9 prevents this cell death.

Apoptosis in Drosophila

In *Drosophila's* wild type embryo, substantial cell death occurs due to apoptosis in a relatively predictable manner. These deaths can be detected in live embryos by staining with vital dyes (*e.g.,*, acridine orange or AO). In 1995, in USA, Hermann Steller and his colleagues identified three overlapping deletions on the third chromosome of *Drosophila,* which abolish all normal or programmed cell deaths. A mutant H99 was later found, which died late in embryogenesis (before hatching) and carried many extra cells in its nervous system. The effect was

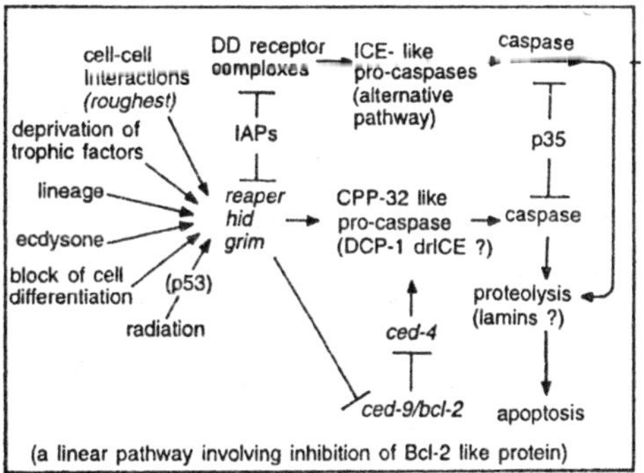

DD = death domain; IAP = inhibitor of apoptosis protein
ICE = interleukin-1β converting enzyme

7 Model for the apoptotic pathway in Drosophila; the genes reaper, hid and grim appear to link many different signaling pathways with the apoptotic programme (redrawn from McCall and Steller, TIG, June 1997).

found to be due to lack of PCD leading to interference with development. It was later shown that this mutant H99 lacked a gene designated as reaper *(rpr)* gene. This reaper *(rpr)* gene plays a central role in apoptosis, so that embryos homozygous for small deletions including *rpr* gene do not exhibit the predictable cell death during embryogenesis. These deletions also protected the embryos against apoptosis caused by X-irradiation and developmental defects.

The apoptosis in these defective embryos could be restored, when the germline was transformed using cloned DNA having *rpr* gene sequences. This reaper *(rpr)* gene is expressed in cells destined to undergo apoptosis as shown by the presence of reaper mRNA and reaper protein (only 65 amino acids long) in these cells. Other genes responsible for morphogenetic cell death due to apoptosis in *Drosophila* are *hid* and *grim,* which link many different signaling pathways with the apoptotic programme (Fig.).

Apoptosis (Cell Death) in Other Cell Systems: The phenomenon of programmed cell death or apoptosis has also been studied in some other animal systems, although not with the same details as done in *Coenorhabditis.* Five systems that have been studied, will be briefly described. These include: (i) metamorphosis in moths; (ii) development of vertebrate neurons, deprived of growth factors; (iii) maturation of mammalian thymocytes, (iv) regression of prostate in rats and (v) programmed cell death in bacterial populations.

Cell Death During Metamorphosis of Moths: In moths, when caterpillar reaches the end of larval stage, it stops feeding and goes underground, to form a pupa, which then develops into an adult. During transition from caterpillar to pupa, most larval muscles die, but intersegmental muscles (in segments A3 to A6) survive. The adult then undergoes ecdysis, shedding unwanted pupal cuticle with the help of surviving intersegmental muscles, which die only after adult ecdysis is complete. Subsequently, some of the neurons that control these muscles also die. Thus at pupal stage, during adult ecdysis and even after adult ecdysis, cells die that are not needed later in the adult. The process of this cell death during metamorphosis in moths has been studied in tobacco hornworm *(Manducta sexta)*, and in giant silkmoth *(Antheraea polyphemus)*.

It has been shown that the same cells always die at a characteristic time during metamorphosis. The timing of these cell deaths is controlled by the steroid hormone, 20-hydroxy -ecdysone, so that the concentration of this hormone declines, when cells are dying and that dying cells can be rescued by injecting this hormone. Besides the levels of this hormone, other factors are also responsible for these cell deaths.

It has also been shown that these deaths of neurons and muscles are suppressed by both actinomycin-D and cycloheximide, suggesting the role of RNA synthesis and protein synthesis in cell death. It means that some novel genes are expressed during cell death. In *Manducta*, a gene encoding polyubiquitin is specially expressed at the time of cell death suggesting the role of polyubiquitin in cell death.

Cell Death of Vertebrate Neurons Deprived of Growth Factors : During the development of vertebrate nervous system, up to 85 per cent of certain populations of neurons undergo cell death, so that this is a striking example of naturally occurring programmed cell death. Following are the two characteristic examples of tissues exhibiting deaths of these neurons in developing chick embryo: (i) the dorsal root sensory ganglia and (ii) the lateral motor column. In each of the these two cases, the number of neurons that die depends upon and is inversely proportional to the size of the target area that these neurons innervate. For instance, if a limb bud is removed, extent of cell death increases (target area to be innervated decreased) and if a supernumerary limb is grafted, the extent of cell death decreases (target area to be innervated increased in this case). This relationship between target area and the extent of cell death suggests that in the target area, there is present a limiting factor, which may regulate cell death. In some neurons this is a 'nerve growth factor' (NGF). Addition of this NGF can prevent cell death *in vitro* and addition of anti-NGF antisera to newborn rodents can increase cell death suggesting that NGF prevents cell death.

However, only certain specific type of neurons respond to NGF. Brain-derived neurotrophic factor (BDNF) and neurotrophin-3 (NT-3) can also promote the survival of embryonic neurons *in vitro* as well as *in vivo*. Both these factors have homology with NGF. There are a number of other factors needed for neuron survival. A 'trophic factor' has been shown to be important in chick embryo. Other proteins include 'ciliary neurotrophic factor (CNTF)' and 'fibroblast growth factors (FGFs)'.

Cell Death of Thymocytes and Mature T-cells: As we know, in mammals, T-cells are involved in providing cellular immunity. Each T-cell type carries a distinct form of T-cell receptor, each of which recognises a specific antigen bound on the surface of another cell, but only in the presence of another protein called major histocompatibility complex (MHC). The immature T-cells called thymocytes, develop in the thymus and have enormous diversity of T-cell receptors. About 95 per cent these thymocytes die before they leave thymus. Most of the thymocytes that die, are those that express inappropriate T-cell receptors, so as to react strongly to cell's own antigens associated with MHC glycoproteins. This helps avoiding autoimmune reactions by negative selection, a process also called clonal deletion.

Programmed cell death of thymocytes is regulated by glucocorticoids, Which induce cell death and act through a steroid receptor. Further, a low level of irradiation and an increased level of cAMP induce cell death, while the growth factors like interleukin-1 and interleukin-2 inhibit cell death. These factors influence cell death indirectly through modulation of the activity of protein kinases to bring about phosphorylation. An endonuclease is also involved in glucocorticoid induced cell death. It causes fragmentation of DNA into fragments 180 bp long (equivalent to the size of a nucleosome). RNA synthesis and protein synthesis is also needed for cell death to occur and may be responsible to maintain sufficient levels of endonuclease, rather than to synthesize another protein essential for cell death to occur.

Mature T cells in the peripheral lymphoid tissue may also be subjected to programmed cell death, if they become autoreactive or autoimmune, due to antigens that were not presented in the thymus. If an immune response is exhibited due to a pathogen, the activated T cells will have to be eliminated after the battle is won, because activated T cells are a potential hazard. The death of such cells due to activation of receptors like Fas, APO-1 and CD95 has recently been demonstrated.

Cell Death in the Regressing Rat Prostate: In male rats, the size of the prostate gland is maintained by a balance between hormone regulated cell death and cell division. In male rats castrated within two weeks after birth, 85 per cent of cells in prostate die leading to reduced size of prostate. On the other hand, if androgens are injected in castrated males, the size of prostate increases due to increased cell division and decreased cell death. Thus most prostate cells are capable of undergoing programmed cell death and the balance between cell death and cell division, is maintained by the level of hormone.

The cell death in prostate resembles changes characteristic of apoptosis and is inhibited by actinomycin D and cyclohexamide suggesting the role of protein synthesis in this cell death. It is also associated with increase in Ca dependent endonuclease activity, which causes DNA fragmentation into pieces 180 bp long. A number of genes also exhibit increased expression during cell death in prostate (*e.g.*, *TRPM-2* gene encoding a protein called 'clusterin').

Programmed Cell Death in Bacterial Populations: According to popular belief, programmed cell death is the characteristic of multicellular organisms and is a part of differentiation and development. Contrary to this belief, in recent years, programmed cell death has also been demonstrated in bacterial cell populations which become heterogeneous due to factors such as cell density, nutrient supply, substratum surface, presence/absence of plasmids incident radiation, viral infection, etc. The passage of time may also account for heterogeneity in bacterial cell populations.

Programmed cell death in some bacterial cell populations has been shown to be caused by the absence of plasmids, so that the cells devoid of plasmids may undergo cell death. The survival of cells with plasmids is facilitated by the presence of a restriction-modification enzyme system, so that the DNA methylases encoded by a plasmid gene provides protection by

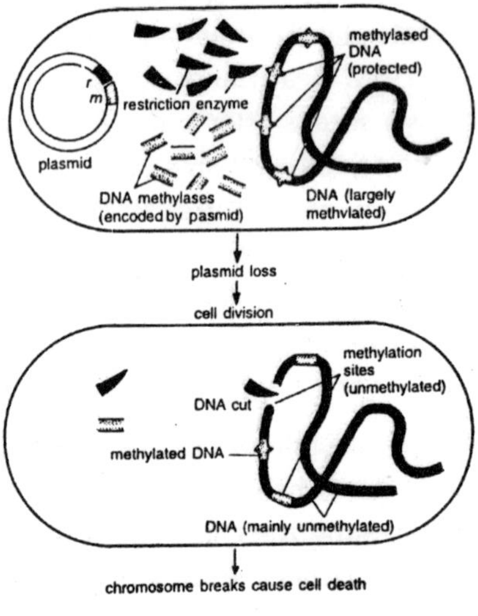

Bacterial death programmed by a plasmid encoded restriction-modification system (redrawn from Yarmolinsy, Science, 10 February, 1995).

methylating the restriction sites. The progeny devoid of a r^+m^+ plasmid (r^+= restriction enzyme gene; m^+=DNA methylase gene) retains insufficient methylase to protect itself from the restriction enzyme so that DNA fragmentation is caused leading to cell death.

Apoptosis (Cell Death) in Cell Cultures: A large number of products are now known to be produced from animal and plant cell cultures. Consequently, considerable efforts are directed towards optimisation of culture conditions for cell growth. Although, considerable cell death takes place in cell cultures, no efforts to control this cell death has been made in the past because it was thought that in culture, cells die by the passive process of necrosis and nothing could be done to control this cell death. However, in recent years, it has been shown that cells die due to experimental stress by a genetically controlled process called apoptosis or PCD and not by simple necrosis (fig.).

Apoptosis in cell cultures can be detected either by examining the morphology of cells (stained with dyes such as haematoxylin) or by extracting and electrophoresing DNA on agarose gels (for detecting internucleosomal DNA fragmentation). Cell shrinkage rather than swelling (as in necrosis) and a ladder of multimeric DNA fragments with a unit of ISObp are two very important parameters used for detection of apoptosis. Flow cytometry based on reduction in DNA staining (due to reduction in binding of dyes) and cell shrinkage is another useful method for detection of apoptosis.

Cells in culture may actually die either by necrosis or by apoptosis. At high stress levels (*e.g.*,, high levels of toxins, sharp changes in pH, high agitation rate, etc.) cells die by necrosis, having no time to respond to the stress. At intermediate level of stress, the cell is injured but not killed so that it can programme its death by apoptosis. At low level of stress, cells can produce heat shock proteins, which enable them to survive until the stress is removed. The death by apoptosis is a safeguard, because such a death does not harm the neighbouring cells, while the death by necrosis does cause injury to the neighbouring cells. Therefore, death by apoptosis is 'cellular friendly' and is a mechanism to overcome stress in culture in a friendly manner.

The cells in culture possess mitogens to drive cell proliferation, and survival factors (*e.g.,*, insulin like growth factor or IGF-1) to prevent apoptosis. The balance between these mitogens and survival factors is important for maintaining high viability in cell cultures. Following two classes of genes are involved in regulation of cell death by apoptosis in cell cultures: (i) genes like *myc* and *p53* driving the process of apoptosis and (ii) genes like *bcl-2, bcr-abl* and *v-abl* inhibiting apoptosis.

Genes that Drive Apoptosis: The genes like *myc* drive both cell proliferation and cell death, depending upon the culture conditions. In the presence of survival signals and Myc protein (encoded by *myc* gene), cells proliferate, and in the absence of survival signals, the cells die by apoptosis. The gene *p53* also causes apoptosis. Following DNA damage, *p53* arrests cells in Gl phase, permitting time for the repair of DNA damage. If DNA damage can not be repaired, apoptosis sets in. If p53 mutates, apoptosis is not triggered and the cell with damaged DNA re-enters the cell cycle causing cancer. In cell cultures, if we wish to limit cell death due to apoptosis, a mutant *p53* may prove useful, although *in vivo* it may prove fatal to the organism. Many cell lines with mutant *p53,* having malignant phenotype have already been developed.

Genes that Inhibit Apoptosis: Genes like *bcl-2* and *bcr-abl,* inhibit apoptosis induced by agents like radiation, serum deprivation and various toxic compounds (Fig.). The mechanism of action of these genes is not quite clear. However, there is some evidence that *bcl-2* may be acting through an anti-oxidant mechanism, where it prevents the apoptotis-inducing effects of reactive oxygen. Other anti-oxidants (*e.g.*, thiocarbamates) have also been shown to inhibit apoptosis, although evidence is also available showing that reactive oxygen may not play a central role in apoptosis signaling pathway. The *bcr-abl* expressing cells are resistant to apoptosis, and the anti-apoptotic property may reside in *abl* portion.

This may lead to increase in tyrosine-kinase activity. Similarly *v-abl* also inhibits apoptosis if transfected into apoptosis sensitive cell lines. Such genes that inhibit apoptosis can be transferred in cell lines producing products of commercial importance, so that the cells will be able to survive short-term sub-optimal conditions. Cell lines that inherently carry these genes do have this property.

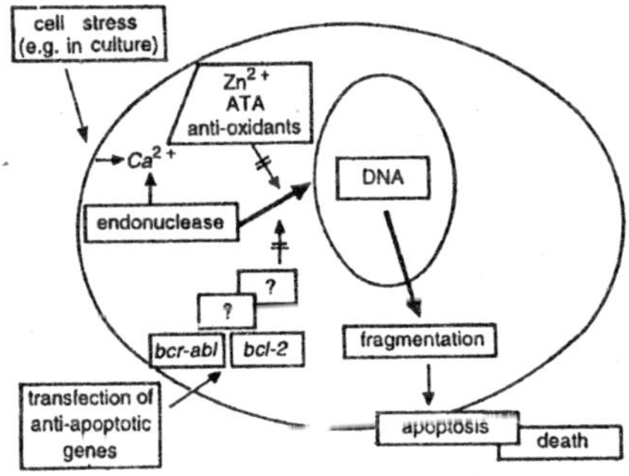

Apoptosis leading to drop in production in cell culture vessels due to environmental stress, and the methods for overcoming this cell death either by transfecting anti-apoptotic genes or by agents like Zn^{2+}, ATA (aurintricarboxylic acid) or by anti-otidants (redrawn from Cotter and Al-Rubeai, TIBTECH, April, 1995).

Culture medium can also be supplemented with survival factors or inhibitors of apoptosis. Compounds like aurintricarboxylic acid (ATA), zinc ions, antioxidants and cytokines are known to inhibit apoptosis. ATA is a nuclease inhibitor and has been shown to inhibit apoptosis without affecting cell proliferation. It is inexpensive and can be used in culture medium to reduce the level of apoptosis.

Objective of Cell Death

Apoptosis or programmed cell death (PCD) is used to kill unwanted cells for the following three purposes: (i) for development and homeostasis ; (ii) for defense and (iii) for aging (senescence). On the basis of the examples of cell death discussed earlier in this chapter, the cells undergoing programmed cell death can be classified in the following five categories: (a) cells having no function; (b) cells that are produced in excess; (c) cells that develop improperly; (d) cells that have finished their function; (e) cells that are harmful and need elimination.

Cells that have no Function: Following are some examples of cells' that die before performing any function: (i) In *C. elegans* many cells die within an hour of their birth, before differentiation starts; (ii) In mammals, many thymocytes die before they mature into T-cells; (iii) In *Manducta* and chick, many cells die at an early stage of neuronal differentiation. In all these cases, why should these cells be produced if they have to die before performing any function? According to one hypothesis, the cells that die before performing any function, are evolutionary vestiges of cells that functioned in an ancestral species. These cell deaths may also facilitate evolutionary changes like the following: (i) While in ducks, there are fewer interdigital cell deaths, so that there is webbing between their toes, in chicken, there is extensive cell death so that the webbing is absent. (ii) Similar cells may divide and undergo divergence due to cell death. For instance, in *C. elegans,* 12 blast cells (P1 to P12) are present along the anterio-posterior axis of young larvae.

Each of these 12 P cells divides and gives one epithelial cell and five different types of motor neurons. In six of the 12 groups of P cell descendants, one or two of the five immature motor neurons die but in the remaining six cells, no cells die. Such a divergence has evolved due to cell death, eliminating neurons that are unnecessary in certain regions of the animal. (iii) In some animal systems, sexual dimorphism evolved due to cell death. For instance, in *C. elegans,* HSN neurons control egg laying in hermaphrodites, but die in males, in which these neurons are unnecessary. Similarly CEM neurons which are responsible for chemotactive movement of males towards hermaphrodites develop in males but die in hermaphrodites. Such examples of the evolution of sexual dimorphism due to cell death are also known in moth *Manducta,* rats, zebra, birds and mammals.

Cells that are Produced in Excess: In *C. elegans,* two male-specific cells (B alapaav and B arapaav) can each form a special part of the proctodeum, needed for mating. Only one of these cells lives and other being in excess die. It has been shown that each of the two cells have the potential to live or die.

Cells that Develop Improperly: The visual system of vertebrates provides with an example, where neurons forming improper connections are eliminated by cell death. In rat, it has been shown that the neurons of the visual system that project their neurons in the wrong region, can be identified by the visual system and are subjected to cell death.

Cells that have Finished their Function: In *C. elegans,* the 'tail- spike cell' generates filaments that help shape the long, tapering tail and then die. Similarly the 'male linker cell' functions during larval development to lead the vas deferens to the cloaca and help it attach, after which this cell dies. Such cell deaths during metamorphosis occur in frog, insects, moths, mammals, etc. (for a review, see Ellis *et.* al., 1991).

Cells that are Harmful: Thymocytes carrying T-cell receptors attacking animal's own tissues (self immunity) are the best example of cells that on maturity injure the animal severely. These are therefore eliminated. Neutrophils is another example of such harmful cells.

Process of Cell Death

As we have seen, programmed cell death or apoptosis is genetically controlled. It is generally regulated by an active process, where specific genes are expressed or enzymes activated to cause cell death (RNA synthesis and protein synthesis must occur for cells to die, although in moths and rats prostate, it could not be demonstrated).

For instance, in *C. elegans, ced-3* and *ced-4* must express within dying cells and Ca^{2+}-dependent endonuclease should be activated to fragment DNA into 180bp pieces. However, there are also mechanisms, which appear to protect cells that should not die due to neighbouring cell death, so that the cell death is a normal process and cell survival is an active process. For instance, in C. *elegans, ced-9* gene and in mammals, *bcl-2* gene appear to be required to prevent many cells from undergoing programmed cell death. Therefore, active processes both for onset of programmed cell death and for preventing this programmed cell death are available in animal cells.

Cell death, whether active process or default state, needs to be studied at the molecular and biochemical level. Only preliminary information from such studies is available, which include the following: (i) Ca^{2+} influx is required for thymocyte death and the deaths of prostate cells; Ca^{2+} ions play an important role in activation of proteins causing cell death. Ca^{2+}-dependent endonuclease is one such example, although Ca^{2+}-independent endonuclease encoded by *nuc'-1* in *C. elegans* also degrades chromosomal DNA, (ii) Protein phosphorylation and de-phosphorylation might also be involved in cell death. For instance, 'protein kinase A' (PKA) is known to induce thymocyte cell death, while 'protein kinase C (PKC) prevents these deaths.

Products of genes like *ced-3* have also been shown to possess phosphorylation sites, suggesting the role of phosphorylation in cell death. Abnormal phosphorylation of cytoskeletal proteins has also been shown to be related to cell deaths during several diseases like 'Alzheimer's's disease', 'Down's syndrome' and 'amyotrophic lateral sclerosis'.

Recently, it has been shown that the control and execution stage of cell death involves interaction between the following

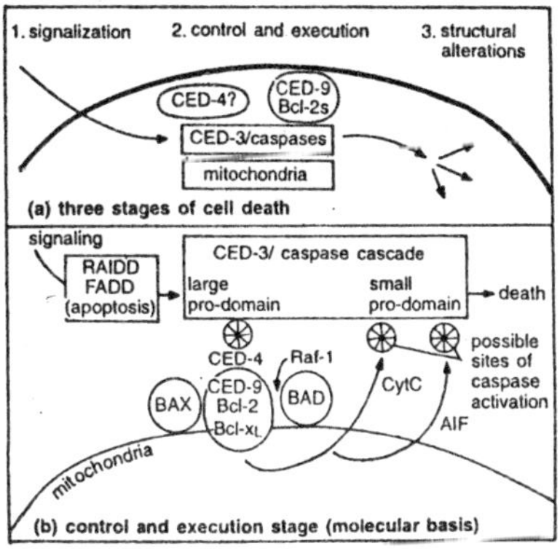

Programmed cell death cascade, depicting the current status of our knowledge about the molecular basis of apoptosis (redrawn from Golstein, Science, 21 February, 1997).

four components: (i) CED-3/caspases, (ii) CED-9/Bcl-2s, (iii) CED-4 and (iv) mitochondria. A connection between Bcl-2 and caspases has been shown to involve CED-4 (product of *ced-4* from *C. elegans*). It has been shown recently that overexpression of CED-4 (homologue of CED-4 in mammals was not discovered till 1997-98), when introduced in mammalian cells, may cause cell death and this cell death can be blocked by overexpression of Bcl-x (homologue of CED-9), and by caspase inhibitors. This suggests that CED-4 is under the control of Bcl-2s and causes death by caspase activation. Physical interaction has also been demonstrated between proteins encoded by *ced-4* and *ced-9* and that between the proteins encoded by *ced-4* and *ced-3* (caspases). It has also been shown that CED-4 can independently or simultaneously bind both CED-9 (Bcl-2) and CED-3 (caspase) so that it eventually forms CED3-CED4-CED9 complexes.

The above interactions seem to take place on mitochondrial membrane and the following scheme seems to be involved (Fig). CED-9/Bcl-2, located at the mitochondrial membrane, binds and modulates CED-4, which in turn binds CED-3/caspases. This leads to caspase activation, if CED-4 is not bound by CED-9/Bcl-2. It also appears that Ref-1 kinase (dragged to mitochondria by Bcl-2) phosphorylates BAD (another member of Bcl-2 family), so that it can not heterodimerise with Bcl-2s thus preventing cell death due to free Bcl-2 (monomers) molecules. Other molecules involved in cell death include the following: (i) Cytochrome-c (Cyt-c) is released from mitochondria and helps in caspase activation, which along with other cytosolic factors, seems to be necessary for cell death. This release of Cyt-c is blocked by Bcl-2. (ii) AIF (apoptosis-inducing factor) is also released from mitochondria and is a 'caspase inhibitor'-sensitive protease, so that it destroys

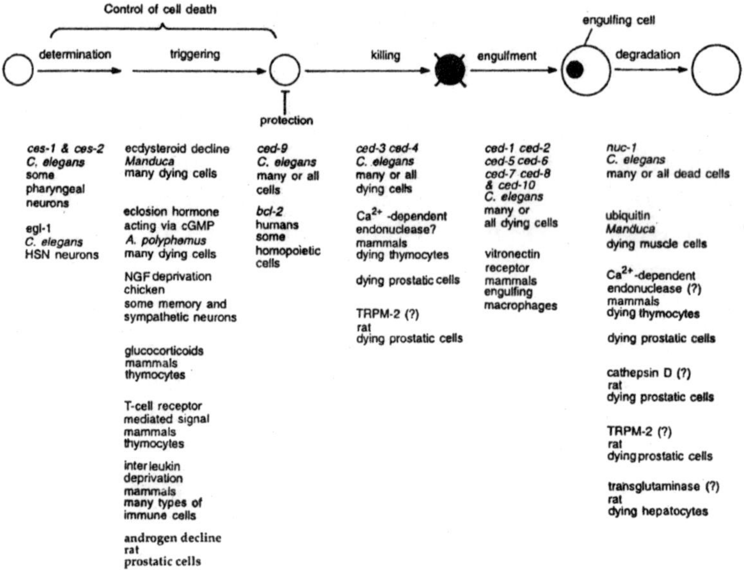

A summary of factors or gene products that act in the process of cell death in C. elegans and in multicellular organisms (redrawn from Ellis et. al., Ann Rev Cell Biol., 1991).

caspase inhibitor and causes caspase activation leading to cell death. Thus there are three links between Bcl-2 and caspase, involving CED-4, Cyt-c and AIF, which may act simultaneously or sequentially .

Another important gene involved in apoptosis in mammals is p53. The p53 protein is a well established activator of one of the pathways to mammalian apoptosis. It has also been shown that p53 perhaps acts by differentially affecting the levels of Bcl-2 and Bax. Recently it has been shown that p53 induced cell death also involves caspase activation, due to release of AIFs, caused by collapse of mitochondrial membrane.

The above information at the molecular level and biochemical level is only very preliminary and fragmented. We still do not know how the different 14 genes responsible for apoptosis in *C. elegans,* act at the molecular level to bring about programmed cell death. The speculated roles of these genes are shown in Figure. More recently (in 1997), proteins called STATs and involved in Jak-STAT pathway, have been shown to be needed for induction of apoptosis due to tumour necrosis factor-α (TNF-a). It has been shown that TNF-α induced apoptosis is defective in mutant cells lacking STATs. This activity of STATs seems to be distinct from their role as cytokine induced transcriptional activators.

Current active research in this area will certainly help in the proper understanding of the mechanism, by which the different genes act and bring about programmed cell death. This information is relevant not only for the study of developmental biology but also in dealing with a variety of diseases caused either due to death of cells that are not supposed to die, or due to survival of cells that were supposed to die. An understanding of cell death may also help us in controlling cancer because an induction of programmed cell death can cause tumour regression.

Apoptosis Targeted Therapies: In order to utilise results of apoptosis research for therapy in human beings, one should understand the mechanism of the regulation of apoptosis in mammalian cells. In May, 1995, a meeting on 'Commercial Prospects of Apoptosis Research' was held in Cambridge, MA (USA). During this meeting it was emphasised that there are three steps in the apoptosis pathway and each step can be either positively regulated towards cell death or negatively regulated towards survival of these cells.

These three steps include the following: (i) The cells for apoptosis are first primed by any of the several kinds of stimuli. The product of the gene p53 (a tumour suppressor gene) may also be one such stimulus meant for priming the cells for apoptosis. (ii) Once the cells are thus primed, in these cells, there is available a brake on death, exercised by survival factor like Bcl-2-Bax heterodimer. This brake has to be released before the processes leading to apoptosis are initiated. (iii) After release of the brake, actual death of cells involving cell shrinkage and chromatin degradation occurs followed by phagocytosis.

In human beings, several diseases may be caused due to apoptosis or lack of it. These may need therapy, keeping in view the information generated from apoptosis research.

Apoptosis in Cells, which should not Die: A disease may result either due to the absence, of some survival factor or due to activation of death genes, which are normally silent in these normal cells. Consequently, therapy for this kind of disease may require either expression or elevation of survival factors or the suppression or inhibition of death genes or their products.

It has recently been shown that Bcl-2 protein or nerve growth factors (NGFs) are actually survival factors rather than inhibitors of apoptosis. In mice, it was shown that if *trkA* gene (gene for NGF receptor) is inactivated; the superior cervical ganglion develops, but soon regresses and disappears, suggesting that NGF or its receptor is a survival factor. In this manner, the survival factors can be used for overcoming unwanted apoptosis. It has also been shown that product of *ced-3* gene in *C. elegans* is homologous to a family of cysteine proteases in mammals, and any inhibitors of cysteine proteases, should therefore be able to inhibit unwanted apoptosis.

ICE (interleukin 1 β converting enzyme) is also a prototype of cysteine proteases, so that the family of these proteases is described as Ich (ICE and ced-3 homology). The inhibitors of the members of Ich family, therefore, can also be utilised for controlling unwanted apoptosis.

The poxvirus gene product (Crm-A) is one such molecule, which specifically inhibits ICE and other members of Ich family. Calpain is yet another cysteine protease that is Ca^{2+} dependent, so that its inhibitor can also be used to block apoptosis. The above information can certainly be useful for developing suitable drugs to control apoptosis.

Following are some examples of unwanted apoptosis, which may need therapeutic treatment as above: (i) In neuroectodermal cells, c-myb levels can be altered by retinoic acid, leading to apoptosis; this may be mediated by the activation of death associated genes, tissue transglutaminase, and other effector elements of cell death (*e.g.*, oxygen and nitric oxide radicals), (ii) Fibroblasts, transfected with *c-myc* gene, grow well in serum containing medium, but undergo rapid per cent apoptosis, if serum is removed; in this system, in the presence of serum, apoptosis is suppressed by growth/ survival factors (*e.g.*, insulin like growth factor or IGF-1) that are present in the serum.

It has also been shown that early tumours sometimes can not grow beyond a certain level (unless there is a second anti-apoptotic mutation), because the supply of survival factors can not keep pace with the growth of the tumours.

Absence of Apoptosis in Cells, which should Die: Apoptosis may sometimes be absent in tissues where death of certain specific cells at a characteristic time is necessary for normal development and differentiation. In these cells destined to die, apoptosis is generally caused by signals transmitted through cell receptors like TNF (tumour necrosis factor) and CD95 (a cytokine). A mutation in CD95 sometimes causes autoimmune disease, so that at least five children were identified during 1994-95, all having autoimmune/lymphoproliferative syndrome. Any successful effort to inhibit the activity of mutant CD95 may cure these children and may eventually lead to the development of a drug for treatment of such syndromes.

Tumours Due to Absence of Normally Occurring Inhibitors of Growth: Tumorous or cancerous growth of cells may also be caused, sometimes due to the absence of normal inhibitors of growth or due to reduced activity of certain normal tumour suppressor genes. In human beings, 50 per cent of the tumours have been shown to have a defective *p53* gene, so that the tumours are more aggressive and are resistant to therapy.

In such tumours, if active p53 gene is introduced, thus increasing the level of p53 protein, the tumours regress. Such a treatment with elevated p53, however, does not do any harm, because this does not lead to any cell death in the normal cells although it does stop growth of tumorous cells. Removal of survival factors can be another method of treating the uncontrolled growth of tumours.

Bibliography

Abbas, A.K, A.H. Lichtman and, J.S. Pober : *Cellular and Molecular Immunology,* Saunders, Philadelphia, 1999.

Ameisen, J. C. : *Tissue Culture,* Oxford, New York, 2000.

Anderson, S. : *Cell Biology,* Oxford University Press, London, 1981.

Atkins, J. F. : *Tissue Culture: an Introduction,* Oxford, New York, 1996.

Auerbach, C. : *Mutation Research: Problems, Results and Perspectives,* Chapman and Hall, London, 2002.

Baker, T.A. : *DNA Replication,* Freeman, New York, 2002.

Beale, G.H. : *Cellular Control Mechanisms and Cancer,* Oxford, New York, 2002.

Becker, W.M. and D.W. Deamer : *The World of the Cell,* Benjamin-Cummings, Redwood City, 2000.

Benjamin, Lewin : *Genes,* Oxford University Press, New York, 2000.

Bennett, R. H. : *Transcription, Processing and Editing in Plant Mitochondria,* Oxford, New York, 1992.

Bittar, E.E. : *Cell Biology in Medicine,* John Wiley, New York, 1999.

Branden, C. and Tooze, J. : *Introduction to Cell Biology,* Garland, New York, 1991.

Court, D. : *Regulatory Sequences Involved in the Promotion and Termination of RNA Transcription,* Cambridge, New York, 2003.

Darnell, J. E. : *Molecular Cell Biology,* Scientific American Books, New York, 1995.

Das, A. : *Control of Transcription Termination,* Routledge, New York, 1993.

Demidov, V. V. : *PNA and LNA throw Light on DNA, Trends,* Oxford, New York, 2003.

DeRobertis, E.D.P. : *Cell Biology,* Waverly Pvt. Ltd., New Delhi, 1988.

DuPraw, E. J. : *Cell and Molecular Biology,* Academic Press, New York, 1969.

Ebby, S. R. : *Non Coding RNA Genes and Modern RNA,* Oxford, New York, 2001

Edlin, G. : *Human Genetics : A Modern Synthesis,* Jones & Bartlett Pub., Boston, 1990.

Ellis, R. J. : *Chloroplast Protein Synthesis,* Oxford, New York, 1975.

Fincham, J.R.S. : *Genetic Complementation,* Benjamin, New York, 1999.

Fournier, M.J. : *The Small Nucleolar RNAs,* MacMillan, London, 1995.

Friedberg, E. C. : *Relationships Between DNA Repair and Transcription,* Oxford, New York, 1996.

Gilbert, W. and B. Muller : *Isolation of the Lac Repressor,* Oxford, New York, 1966.

Gilham, N. W. : *Genetic Analysis of the Chloroplast and Mitochondrial Genomes,* Oxford, New York, 1974.

Glick, B. and G. Schatz : *Import of Proteins into Mitochondria,* Oxford, New York, 1991.

Gray, M. W. : *The Evolutionary Origin of Organelles*, Oxford, New York, 1989.

Grunstein, M. : *Histones as Regulators of Genes*, Oxford, New York, 1992.

Gupta, P. K. : *Cell Biology*, Rastogi Publications, Meerut, 2000.

Hadjiolov, A. A. : *The Nucleolus and Ribosome Biogenesis*, Oxford, New York, 1985.

Henikoff, S. : *Cell Biology : A Reference Manual*, MIT Press, Cambridge, 2002.

Hoagland, M. G. : *The Present Status of the Adaptor Hypothesis*, MacMillan, London, 1959.

Holley, R. W. : *Structure of a Ribonucleic Acid*, McGraw Hill, London, 2002.

Hunt, T. : *The Cell Cycle*, Oxford University Press, Oxford, 2002.

Ingram, V. : *The Biosynthesis of Macromolecules*, Benjamin, New York, 2001.

Jacobson, M. : *Developmental Neurobiology*, Plenum Press, New York, 2002.

Jukes, T. H. : *Mitochondrial Codes and Evolution*, Oxford, New York, 2000.

Kaguni, L. S. : *Eukaryotic DNA Polymerase-primase : Structure, Mechanism and Function*, MacMillan, London, 1999.

Kaziro, Y: *Structure and Function of Signal Transducing GTP Binding Proteins*, Blackwell, London, 2001.

Kendrew, J. C. : *The Three-dimensional Structure of a Protein Molecule*, Sinauer, New York, 1991

Kramer, A. :*The Structure and Function of Proteins Involved in Mammalian Pre-mRNA Splicing*, Grandada, New York, 2001.

Kurland, C. G. : *Structure and Function of the Bacterial Ribosomes*, Oxford, New York, 2000.

Lehninger, A. L. : *Cell Biology*, Academic Press, New York, 2001

McKnight, S. L. : *Molecular Zippers in Gene Regulation*, Princeton, New York, 2002.

Merrick, W. C. : *Overview : Mechanism of Translation Initiation in Eukaryotes*, Longman, London, 2001.

Moore, P. B. : *Molecular Mimicry in Protein Synthesis*, Cambridge, London, 2002.

Noller, H. F. : *Ribosomol RNA and Translation*, Oxford, New York, 1999.

Olson, R. E. : *Enzymatic Synthesis of DNA*, John Wiley, New York, 2001.

Owen, L. : *DNA Synthesis*, Freeeman, San Francisco, 2001.

Pardee, A. B. : *Molecular Basis of Biological Regulation: Origins of Feedback Inhibition and Allostery*, Arnold, London, 2003.

Paszkowski, J. : *DNA and Histone Methylation in Plants*, MacMillan, London, 2002.

Razin, A. and A. D. Riggs : *DNA Methylation and Gene Function*, Longman, New York, 2002.

Reinbcrg, D. : *Common Themes in Assembly and Function of Eukaryotic Transcription Complexes*, MacMillan, London, 2002.

Rich, A. and S. H. Kim : *The Three Dimensional Structure of Transfer RNA*, Oxford, New York, 1999.

Robertson, M. : *RNA Processing : the Post-RNA World*, Oxford, New York, 1999.

Sauer, R. T. : *Transcription Factors : Structural Families and Principles of DNA Recognition*, Printice Hall, London, 1993.

Schmid, M. B. : *Structure and Function of the Bacterial Chromosome*, Granada, London, 1990.

Stryer, L. : *Cell Biology*, W.H. Freeman & Co., New York, 2002.

Temin, H. M. : *RNA Directed DNA Synthesis,* MacGraw-Hill, New York, 2002.

Threadgold, L.T. : *The Infrastructure of Animal Cell,* Pergamon Press, London, 1999.

Turner, B. M. : *Histone Acetylation and Control of Gene Expression,* MacMillan, London, 2002.

Ulrich, B. : *Mechanism and Regulation of Eukaryotic Protein Synthesis,* Oxford, New York, 2002.

Uptain, S. M. : *Basic Mechanisms of Transcript Elongation and its Regulation,* MacMillan, London, 1997.

Voinnet, O. : *RNA Silencing : Small RNAs as Ubiquitous Regulators of Gene Expression,* MacMillan, London, 2002.

Walbot, V. : *Structure of Plant Mitochondrial Genomes,* John Wiley, London, 1992.

Wallace, D. C. : *Diseases of the Mitochondrial DNA,* Blackwell, New York, 2002.

Wang, T. S. F. : *Eukaryotic DNA Polymerases,* MacMillan, London, 2002.

Wilkins, M. H. F. : *Physical Studies of the Molecular Structure of Deoxyribose Nucleic Acid and Nucleoprotein,* MacMillan, London, 2002.

Woese, C. R. : *The Genetic Code : The Molecular Basis for Genetic Expression,* Harper & Row, New York, 2003.

Wuthrich, K. : *A Hand Book of Cell Biology,* Oxford, New York, 2001.

Yanofsky, C. : *Introduction Tissue Culture,* Oxford, New York, 2001.

Yarus, M. : *Translational Efficiency of Transfer RNAs,* Oxford, New York, 2002.

Zetka, M. : *History of Tissue Culture,* Oxford, New York, 2002.

Index

D

E

F

G

H

N

O

P

R

❑❑❑